Waxing Made Easy:
A Step-by-Step Guide

DETROIT
PUBLIC
LIBRARY

D0166821

Waxing Made Easy:

A Step-by-Step Guide

Renée Poignard

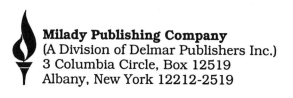

Milady Publishing Company
(A Division of Delmar Publishers Inc.)
3 Columbia Circle, Box 12519
Albany, New York 12212-2519

NOTICE TO THE READER

Publisher does not warrant or guarantee any of the products described herein or perform any independent analysis in connection with any of the product information contained herein. Publisher does not assume, and expressly disclaims, any obligation to obtain and include information other than that provided to it by the manufacturer.

The reader is expressly warned to consider and adopt all safety precautions that might be indicated by the activities described herein and to avoid all potential hazards. By following the instructions contained herein, the reader willingly assumes all risks in connection with such instructions.

The publisher makes no representations or warranties of any kind, including but not limited to, the warranties of fitness for particular purpose or merchantability, nor are any such representations implied with respect to the material set forth herein, and the publisher takes no responsibility with respect to such material. The publisher shall not be liable for any special, consequential or exemplary damages resulting, in whole or in part, from the readers' use of, or reliance upon, this material.

Credits:
Publisher: Catherine Frangie
Editorial Assistant: Amy Clinton
Senior Project Editor: Laura Miller
Freelance Project Editor: Pamela Fuller
Production Manager: John Mickelbank
Art Supervisor: Susan Mathews

Photos courtesy Marvin G. Turner, Golden Moon Productions

Copyright © 1994
Milady Publishing Company
(A Division of Delmar Publishers Inc).

Printed in the United States of America
Published simultaneously in Canada
by Nelson Canada
a division of The Thomson Corporation

1 2 3 4 5 6 7 8 9 10 XXX 00 99 98 97 96 95 94

Library of Congress Cataloging-in-Publication Data

Poignard, Renée.
    Waxing made easy: a step-by-step guide/Renée Poignard.
        p.   cm.
    ISBN 1-56253-171-9
    1. Hair—Removal.   I. Title.
RL92.P65   1994
646.7'24—dc20

                                                    93-25343
                                                    CIP

To Rozelle for unrelentless dedication, support, and patience. Janie, thank you for taking the time to show me how.

Table of Contents

CHAPTER SIX

CHAPTER SEVEN

Introduction

A client came into a salon for facial services and mentioned that she was going to see Halley's Comet in South America. I asked her if she needed any services for the trip. I mentioned lash dying, brow shaping, and hair removal. She said, "I would like to have a bikini wax, but I don't have enough time for the bruising and soreness to go away." I asked, "What bruising and soreness?" She explained that after waxing you bruise, and that the area is very tender for a couple of days before you can put on a bathing suit. I spent quite a few minutes explaining to her that bruising is not necessary if you use proper waxing techniques. The only way I could convince her was to give her the service for no charge, with my word that everything would be fine. After the waxing service she couldn't believe that it had been so simple, quick, and painless!

Many clients have told me similar stories about their waxing experiences. There is no need for waxing sessions to turn out bad and ruin your reputation as an epilator. I think that all potential epilators should ask themselves this question before beginning to wax a client: "Do you enjoy waxing or do you find it a burden—messy, frustrating, and time consuming?" If your answer is that you enjoy it, you will find this manual useful. The helpful tips and waxing techniques will help eliminate most frustrations that occur with waxing and will help you develop waxing skills that will earn you praise. This manual is designed for those new to epilation, but experienced epilators will find new methods, remedies for existing problems, and added knowledge.

Waxing can be a rewarding part of your esthetic experience. It can be financially rewarding, especially during the summer months. It can also provide a boost in your career, because you will feel great when clients compliment your exceptionally good skills.

To become an elite epilator I encourage you to study the information provided in this manual. I encourage you to take your time in learning the practical applications. I advise you to find a licensed practicing epilator who will allow you to observe procedures. (This will enable you to recognize the techniques mentioned in the manual and thereby strengthen your abilities to use them.)

Last, I encourage you to strive for perfection! To become a perfectionist means nothing is left undone. Every hair is removed, and your client understands any further actions you are going to take to correct future problems. Please take a deep breath, relax, read the material, apply the techniques, review your work, assess your errors, make proper corrections, and realize that practice does make perfect!

I often think of how wonderful it would be to have a salon that specializes in hair removal. The salon would include electrolysis, tweezing, and waxing. The reason I think this type of salon would do very well is that the demand for waxing is increasing. The summer months is a good time to increase your waxing business. Waxing is a great giveaway to introduce hair-removal services to your clients. Waxing can help you financially. If you offer hair care, facials, and massages, you can increase your service ticket by observing your clients. When you're working with a client, ask yourself these questions. "Does my client have hair around her mouth?" "Will a proper brow shape give my client a more youthful look?" "Can my client benefit from a bathing suit waxing for vacation?"

If you have good waxing skills, you can be assured of a good increase in business if you observe your clients and sell your services. Word travels very quickly when there is a good epilator in the neighborhood.

CHAPTER ONE

Understanding Depilatory Waxing

CHAPTER OBJECTIVES

1. To understand why depilatory waxing is so popular
2. To be able to draw and label the hair follicle and shaft
3. To understand some of the factors to be considered before choosing electrolysis

A client came for the first time to a skin-care salon for hair removal services. The esthetician noticed that she seemed a little shy and somewhat hesitant. The esthetician explained the procedure of depilatory waxing and then performed the service. When it was over, the client looked in the mirror and began to cry. She explained that earlier in the day she had found a shaving mug, brush, and razor on her desk. Someone had found a cruel way of telling her to remove the hair from her lips and chin. The client said it had always been a problem and that she had thought there was no solution. She didn't know that most women experience unwanted hair in those areas. She also said that if she had known there were services like waxing she would have had the hair removed years ago.

Many women who have unwanted hair do not know about depilatory waxing. Waxing is not a new art—

hair removal by waxing has been popular since ancient times. It is popular because it is quick, simple, convenient, and affordable. Let's review all the methods of hair removal and find out why many client and professionals prefer waxing over other methods.

Understanding the Hair and Its Structure

The hair is a slender, thread-like outgrowth of the skin and scalp. It is composed of keratin. The tough, elastic material forms sheets of long, endless fibers, and it does not normally break off or flake away. The hair develops within a sheath called a follicle. New hairs are formed from cells at the bottom of the follicle. At the bottom of the follicle is the papilla, which is the base where the blood supplies nourishment to the cells and forms new hairs. Attached to most hair follicles is a thin band of involuntary muscles. As the muscle contracts it presses on the sebaceous gland, attached to the hair follicle, causing the release of sebum to lubricate the skin. Every inch of skin contains 1,300 nerve endings to record pain. The importance of these three factors—involuntary muscles, nerve endings, and sebaceous glands—will be explained later in chapter 4.

Hair Removal Methods

Unwanted hair can be removed in a number of ways—some more effective than others. The following methods are those that are most often used.

Shaving

The most common and probably the most widely used method of hair removal is shaving. Shaving is simple, easy, and convenient. A sharp razor is glided over the skin, and hair is removed (Figures 1–1 and 1–2). There are several disadvantages of shaving, especially for areas of the body that are usually exposed (brows, lips, chins, and arms). First, since shaving only removes the hair topically, hair regrowth is rapid. Some hair begins to grow back the same day or the next. Second, in sensitive areas, like the bikini line area, the chin, and the sides of the face, bumping can occur. This usually hap-

FIGURE 1–1
Lotion is applied to the hair before shaving.

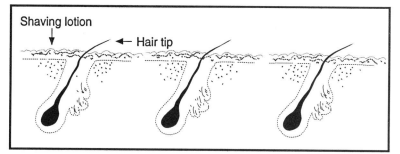

FIGURE 1–2
A sharp razor is drawn over the skin, and hair is removed.

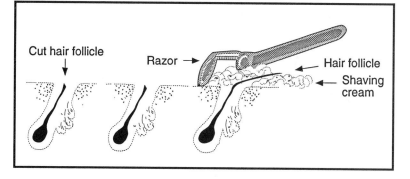

FIGURE 1–3
During shaving the hair is cut bluntly.

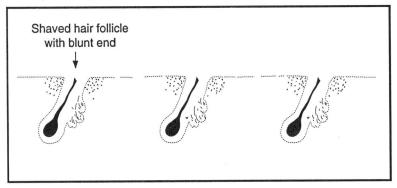

Shaved hair follicle
with blunt end

pens when the end of the hair follicle is cut off bluntly
(Figure 1–3). This blunt edge has to force itself
through a fine pore, which is designed for the entry of
an almost invisible fine tip of hair. Forcing a blunt
edge through a fine pore can cause irritation in the
form of a papule (bump) (Figure 1–4). Another short-
coming of shaving is that in some cases the fine pieces
of cut hair (Figure 1–5) fall back into the now empty

FIGURE 1–4
Bumping can occur when
the blunt hair forces itself
through the follicle.

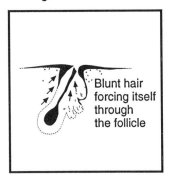

Blunt hair
forcing itself
through
the follicle

FIGURE 1–5
Fine pieces of cut hair can
fall back into the empty
shaft.

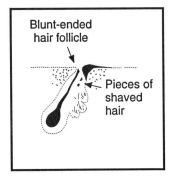

Blunt-ended
hair follicle

Pieces of
shaved
hair

FIGURE 1–6
An infection, or pustice, can be caused by pieces of hair caught in the follicle.

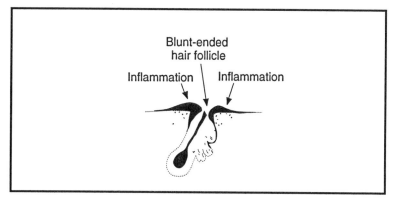

shaft, causing an infection in the form of a pustule (Figure 1-6). If a hair follicle grows out and curls back into the skin (pseudofolliculitis), shaving is most irritating. In order to remove hair closely, the razor blade must be sharp. A sharp blade removes not only hair but also dead skin cells. The daily removal of dead skin cells can break down the skin barrier, which causes sensitivity in some people.

Tweezing

Tweezing is a method of hair removal used to remove undesired hair from eyebrows, chin, and around the mouth (Figure 1–7). Normally tweezing is used to remove one or two undesirable hairs (Figure 1–8). Tweezing is not used for larger areas because it is too time consuming. Tweezing too many hairs at a time increases the chance of breaking the hair below the skin's surface (Figure 1–9). Breaking the hair in the hair shaft will cause rapid regrowth and irritation from the blunt tip.

FIGURE 1–7
Tweezing is another method of removing unwanted hairs.

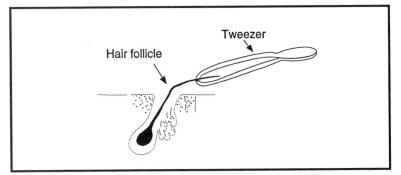

FIGURE 1–8
Normally one or two hairs are tweezed at a time.

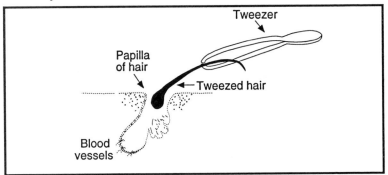

FIGURE 1–9
Tweezing too many hairs at once, or improper use of tweezers, increases breakage.

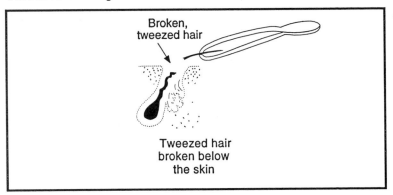

Chemical Depilatory

Chemical depilatories are available in the form of cream, paste, or powder (Figure 1–10). Depilatories are used to remove hair from legs, bikini areas, and underarms (Figure 1–11). The hair is removed when the depilatory solution is washed away from the skin's surface (Figure 1–12). This method of hair removal results in rapid regrowth and the loss of the skin's barrier. The skin becomes irritated and sensitive when a second chemical solution is applied. It makes sense that a chemical that can dissolve hard keratin could be too strong for the average skin. The most common complaints about chemical depilatories are that they

FIGURE 1–10
Chemical depilatories come in the forms of cream, paste, or powder.

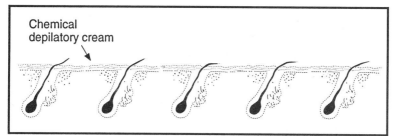

FIGURE 1–11
Chemical depilatories are used to remove hair from the legs, bikini area, and underarms.

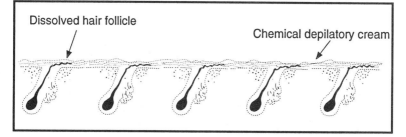

FIGURE 1–12
Hair is removed when the depilatory solution is washed away from the skin's surface.

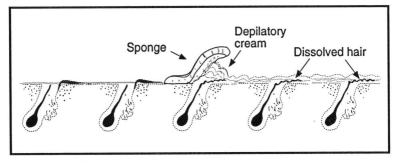

leave chemical burns, tenderness, and small cysts, so when you need to reapply you cannot always do so.

Electrolysis

Electrolysis is thought of as a permanent means of hair removal. When electrolysis is used, the papilla, which supplies nourishment to the hair, is destroyed. An electrolysis practitioner should be certified and well trained before practicing hair removal with electricity. Different methods are used in electrolysis. The three methods are galvanic, short-wave, and the blend method. A needle is angled along the side of the hair follicle to the hair root, and a current is applied (Figure 1–13). A tweezer is then used to remove the hair and its coagulated papilla (Figure 1–14). Electrolysis is recommended for the client with excessive undesired hair. Electrolysis seems to be a good choice for hair removal, but certain factors should be considered. First, it is a very uncomfortable procedure. It could take one to three years or longer to permanently destroy the hair from large areas. The cost of electrolysis can be quite high. The cost is based on how many hairs are removed. The charge for each hair ranges from one to

FIGURE 1–13
A needle is inserted into the hair follicle, and a current is applied.

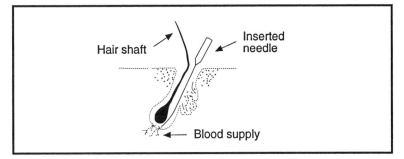

FIGURE 1–14
A tweezer is used to remove hair and its coagulated papilla.

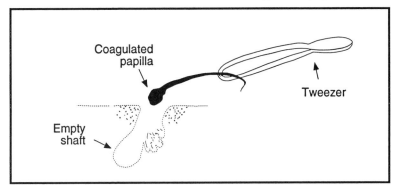

two dollars. An experienced electrologist can remove one hair in thirty seconds, so the client can have as many as two hairs removed in each minute. The cost could be thirty to sixty dollars for thirty minutes of service. However, the permanent result may outweigh the expense.

Physical Depilatory (Waxing)

Soft waxing is rapidly becoming the most accepted means of hair removal. In depilatory waxing, a thin

FIGURE 1–15

A soft layer of wax is spread on the skin.

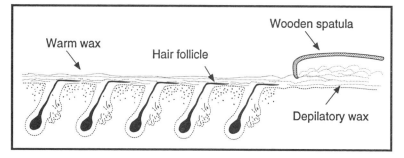

layer of soft wax is applied (Figure 1–15), then pulled against the direction of the hair growth (Figure 1–16). The benefits of depilatory waxing are many. First, it is ideal for any size area. It is highly recommended for sensitive and delicate areas. All the hair in one area can be removed in one visit, from the top of the head to the tip of the toes. Waxing is easy, convenient, and quick. An experienced epilator can wax a set of lower legs in less than twenty minutes. Waxing causes some temporary discomfort. The cost for the hair removal

FIGURE 1–16

Muslin is used to remove wax and hair by pulling in the opposite direction of hair growth.

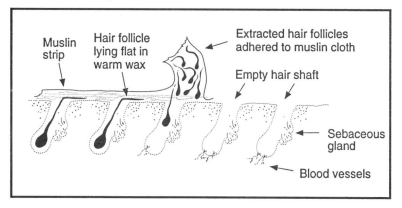

service is reasonable and affordable. The materials needed to wax cost only pennies—the client is actually paying for the epilator's time and expertise. Along with removing the hair, the waxing also removes just the right number of dead skin cells. The removal of the cells by waxing leaves the skin soft and smooth. An additional benefit of waxing is that it takes four to six weeks before a new cycle of hair comes to the surface. The comments of clients who have received depilatory waxing over a period of one to two years can be summarized: "the hair grows back sparsely, softly, and less quickly and I feel cleaner, fresher, and healthier."

We have discussed several common means of hair removal. This information can be used by you when you talk to clients who have expressed interest in waxing. Remember, never slander another hair removal service or a client's choice. Encourage and guide your clients about the practical benefits of waxing.

REVIEW QUESTIONS

1. Why is depilatory waxing so popular?
2. In addition to depilatory waxing, what are some other methods of hair removal?
3. Describe the structure of the hair.
4. What are some factors a client must consider before choosing electrolysis?

C H A P T E R
T W O

Materials Needed for Waxing

CHAPTER OBJECTIVES

1. To introduce the epilator to different kinds of waxes

2. To list various kinds of waxing strips and the sizes needed for waxing different areas

3. To discuss different types of spatulas and their uses

4. To discuss the advantages of disposable products

5. To show different prewax products and the advantages of using them

Depilatory Waxes

Many different commercial brands of depilatory wax are on the market today. The important variables are the texture and the type of resin that is used in waxes. The texture of wax can be determined once the wax is heated. Some epilators like their wax to be thick, while others prefer it to be thin. On the market today manufacturers are being innovative in improving the quality of the wax base. Resin is the substance that gives the wax its texture. A gum resin base can cause sensitivity in some clients. To overcome this problem manufacturers have added essential oils like azulene to aid in calming the skin. Other manufacturers have entirely changed the base of the waxes so the customer won't experience sensitivity. The most common waxes are made of honey wax. I have, however, seen waxes that have the texture and hue of satin paint. I can only advise the epilator to experience the different choices on the market today, and to evaluate the texture, smell, required heating, and cost when choosing a wax.

Cold wax requires a separate heating element; manufacturers offer cold wax heaters. Cold wax does not require as high a temperature as honey wax. Cold wax is used without muslin strips, and is generally used for waxing facial areas. However, one wax, called "green wax," is used for the leg, bikini area, and arms. This wax doesn't cool as quickly, and the texture is more like that of the honey wax. If the cold wax cools before it is removed it can dry hard, which makes it difficult to remove. Cold wax comes in many different forms, including a small sectioned block, the shape of beads, and in the same containers as that of honey wax.

Muslin Cloth

Most wax manufacturers carry a brand of muslin cloth. It can be woven or of a muslin texture, which is referred to as nonwoven. Manufacturers offer precut strips of muslin cloth that can be cut to wax legs or can be cut to fit smaller areas. One manufacturer markets a wax that requires the use of cellophane. Test the different types of cloth and decide which is better for your services. One of the most economical ways to purchase muslin is to buy it in bulk by the yard. Cloth stores carry muslin. When you are purchasing muslin, request muslin that has not been treated with a fabric softener. Unbleached muslin is best. Place your hand under the muslin; if you can see your hand through the material, it is too thin. You do not want to get a piece that is too thick, either. The best way to judge is to take a commercial brand of muslin with you to compare. The muslin sizes needed to wax specific areas are as follows, lip: 1 $\frac{1}{2}$ by 4 inches; brow: 1 $\frac{1}{2}$ by 4 inches; chin: 2 by 2 inches; underarms: 3 by 6 inches; arms: 3 $\frac{1}{2}$ by 6 inches; legs: 4 by 9 inches.

Spatulas

Tongue suppressors are commonly used in waxing, although many different types of instruments can be used. I would first read the rules of the State Cosmetology Board to be sure to follow their requirements. Tongue suppressors are most commonly used because you can dispose of them after their use. They can be cut to fit your needs. When waxing the lip or brow you can cut the tongue suppressor in thirds. For waxing chins or underarms you can cut the tongue suppressor in half (Figure 2-1). You should trim the tongue suppressor to fit your personal needs.

Teakwood spatulas are becoming popular. The reason for this popularity is that they can be used over and over again (Figure 2-2). The teakwood is polished to a high gloss, which prevents the wood from absorbing any scents, liquids, or bacteria. You can also disinfect the teakwood as well as sterilize it. Another reason teakwood is so popular is that a variety of sizes are available to fit the needs of waxing. An example of this is the spatula used for waxing legs; it is 10 to 12 inches long and 2 inches wide. Today you will find on the market Teflon coated spatulas, plastic spatulas, and stainless steel spatulas, and I'm quite sure there are many more, of all shapes, colors, and textures. I suggest you try several until you find the size and type suitable for your needs.

FIGURE 2–1

For waxing chins and underarms, cut the tongue suppressor to half its size.

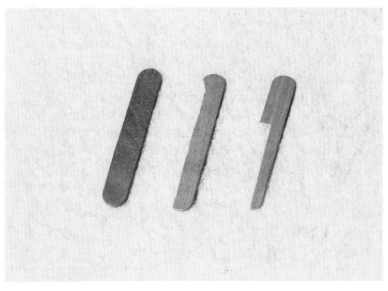

FIGURE 2–2

Teakwood spatulas are popular.

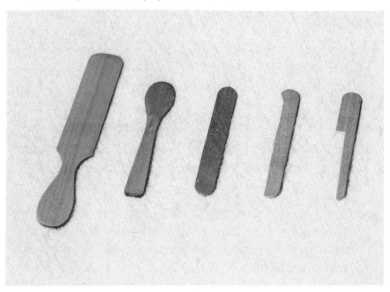

Disposable Paper Goods

On the market today are several types of paper goods designed to help the epilator. The most commonly used is roll paper, which protects the waxing table. A waxing cloth is available that is prepared like sheets. This material is very comfortable for the client. The cost is usually much higher than that of rolled paper. Disposable bikinis are becoming more popular for the epilator. Clients can put them on and discard them after waxing. Paper vests are available for the client to wear to protect the clothing from possible wax spills. Some epilators are using face masks when waxing certain areas of the body for sanitation reasons.

Waxing Lotions

Creams, oils, gels, pastes, and powders are all different forms of skin conditioners. Usually depilatory wax manufacturers offer a line of products to aid in waxing.

Prewaxing lotions are designed to clean the area before waxing. You can use your good judgment about whether this product should be used for a particular service.

Powder is used to absorb oils and moisture, and some claim it lessens the client's discomfort. Again, it is the epilator's personal decision when and if there is a need for powder.

Antiseptics are used after a waxing procedure. This helps to soothe the skin, cleanse the area, and prevent possible skin irritation. Slow growth products are used after the antiseptics to fill the hair follicle shaft. These products have not been proven in the laboratory, but clients say they notice their effect on particular hair growth.

Afterwax products are used to calm the skin as well as to take the redness out. One such product actually contains menthol and is colored beige to mask the redness. Essential oil base afterwax products come with Dr. Jock's Wort Oil, menthol, cloves, lavender, camomile, and many other additives. All varieties are designed to calm the skin and take out redness.

The market is saturated with products to aid the epilator. I suggest you try several until you find the products that give you the best results.

Wax Heaters

Salon equipment manufacturers sell wax heaters. Most heaters have regulators that allow you to adjust the wax temperature. The more wax the heater processes, the more expensive it will be. When you are shopping for a heater, look for the following qualities. (1) The most important variable is the heat regulator. Some heaters have high, medium, and low settings. A good heater will have a thermostat that can be adjusted to all levels, from 60 to 130 degrees. The thermostat should be able to regulate itself, so that when the unit reaches the desired temperature it will turn itself off. When the temperature drops below the desired level it will turn itself on. This will prevent the wax from burning. (2) A stainless steel basket insert. This basket will make it easy to clean the waxer. Any foreign objects that fall into the wax can be retrieved by lifting the basket. (3) A stainless steel or metal container. This will help you clean the wax pot with ease. Sometimes plastic containers are difficult to clean, and thus become less attractive. (4) It would be wonderful to have a container collar made of stainless steel and designed to prevent spillage. Otherwise manufacturers do make paper collars. (5) The capacity to hold several cans of wax. I suggest a facial wax heater designed for one can of wax. I also suggest a larger container that will hold three to five cans of wax for the waxing room.

A popular heating element that is simple to use is a disposable wax container. The wax is stored in a plastic container that fits a heating element. The containers come in different sizes. Once the container is empty, the epilator throws it away and replaces it with a new plastic container.

The epilator has many choices of products, materials, and heating elements. A visit to a skin-care convention will give you the opportunity to see, touch, smell, and try all those available to you, so I suggest you attend the next time a convention is available.

REVIEW QUESTIONS

1. What is the purpose of prewax products?
2. What is the difference between soft wax and cold wax?
3. What is the suggested size for brow, chin, and leg strips?
4. Why should disposable products be considered?
5. What product is considered the most practical spatula?

THREE

Sanitation and Sterilization

CHAPTER OBJECTIVES

1. To discuss correct disinfection and sterilization procedures for waxing implements

2. To familiarize the epilator with where to go to find out the state's sanitation and sterilization regulations

3. To emphasize the importance of wearing gloves during the waxing procedure

A client came to me once for waxing services. While we were going through the procedure she mentioned that she used to go to a salon several blocks away from me. When she learned that I was doing waxing services, she booked her next appointment with me. I asked her why she wasn't pleased with her epilator. She said that she liked the way the epilator waxed; however, the wax room was always dirty, and the client felt unsafe. She also mentioned that the epilator had asked her where she had been since she hadn't seen her in a while. The client told her that she was using a salon closer to her home. The client never mentioned the unsanitary conditions. Clients will leave your services, go somewhere else, and never mention that your salon is dirty. Make sure that clients you haven't seen for a while did not leave because your salon isn't kept clean and neat. Some reputations are hard to correct.

Today, more than ever, people are concerned about the health status of individuals serving the public as well as those receiving services. Many beauty professionals are faced with decisions that never were a concern before. Should gloves be worn during services? Does my disinfectant cover all bacteria present today? Is a face mask really necessary to perform certain treatments? These are the rules, regulations, and concerns that should be discussed in the beauty profession today regarding sterilization and sanitation techniques. We will discuss a few and how they affect the epilator.

Practices That Promote Good Sanitation

Each state has a governing body that regulates the beauty profession. You should send for the rules and regulations set by your particular state. You should contact a distributor who carries a variety of products designed to destroy bacteria. You should invest in disposable goods, which help protect clients, bedding, and help eliminate the possibility of spreading germs.

You should make a vow to clean up after every client, change the linen, dispose of all used items, faithfully strip down the waxing area, and thoroughly clean and disinfect every surface at least once a week. Daily cleansing of all instruments and cleaning the work area after each client are musts. You must remember to wash your hands after each client with a bacteria-killing soap.

Cleaning Instruments

Cleaning instruments is simple. Each implement should be washed with a bacteria-killing soap. Then the implements should be immersed in a disinfectant solution (Barbicide, Formalin, alcohol) for at least twenty minutes, then stored in a sterilizer or a storage cabinet containing Formalin tablets.

Linen should be cleaned with bleach. Disposable paper should be used to protect sheets during waxing. All linen should be kept in a storage cabinet. Wax can be very messy, so protect your linen with disposable sheets. It will also give the wax room a more clinical appearance.

Containers, wax heaters, and the wax table can become very soiled with wax. Every day I would encourage you to take the time to clean. If the wax residue is allowed to build up, cleaning becomes more difficult. One item I have found to be useful for the epilator is freezer paper. The paper is white, so it looks clinical. The underside of the paper is waxed, so it can protect your table and any other item that needs to be protected from wax. Oil is very effective for removing wax residue from instruments, tables, and wax heaters. Again, it is good for removing wax residue, but only on the items mentioned above. Oil and petroleum jelly are not designed to remove wax from the skin.

Gloves

Should you wear gloves, or not? This decision should be yours. Often when you are waxing blood appears. This poses a problem for many epilators. Remember, the best protection against exposing yourself to bacteria is your own unbroken skin. If your skin is unbroken, harmful germs cannot enter. If you do have cuts in your skin, you may want to wear gloves. On the market today are several products designed to protect the hands. They are referred to as liquid gloves. They protect the hands as long as they are not washed. Using alcohol before you wax and after you wash your hands offers some protection. The decision of whether and when to wear gloves is the personal choice of each epilator. Use your judgment to decide whether the gloves are needed.

The most important advice I could give is to keep the wax area clean. Stop and ask yourself, would you be comfortable removing your clothing and lying on your bed? Would you be willing to lay your head on the head support? If you look at your wax heater and implements, would you want them used on your face or on private areas of your body? If you can answer yes, then you will increase your clientele base with a good, clean reputation.

REVIEW QUESTIONS

1. What source should the epilator turn to for sterilization and sanitation requirements?
2. Why should the epilator wear gloves?
3. What is the best way to sterilize implements?
4. What should the epilator's attitude be about maintaining the facility?

FOUR

Waxing Procedures, Techniques, and Helpful Hints

CHAPTER OBJECTIVES

1. To show the epilator how to determine the correct wax temperature

2. To show the importance and the method of controlling wax

3. To discuss basic waxing steps

This chapter will help the new epilator understand waxing techniques, which will help make learning depilatory waxing easier. The helpful hints will aid all those who need assistance in improving their waxing technique.

There was a very artistic esthetician who had excellent skills, with the exception of waxing. After a waxing service, the esthetician would think, "I hate waxing." The esthetician would think this while removing wax from hands, clothes, floor, and wax equipment. The esthetician didn't realize that every client felt the same way. The clients usually experienced burns or bruising, or spent the rest of the day trying to remove the wax residue. Fortunately, a coworker took the time to watch the esthetician wax. The experienced epilator told her, "All you need to know is the proper waxing procedure and a few waxing tips." In one day the es-

23

thetician learned proper waxing, and within a few weeks her waxing services were being requested. The esthetician's response to why there was a big change: "Someone just had to tell me how!" So now I am passing those waxing tips on to you.

Depilatory waxing is simple and easy. If you learn the basic concepts and techniques of waxing, you will find yourself performing waxing services with ease.

The basic concepts behind waxing can be applied to any area, no matter how large or small. The techniques given in this chapter should help you eliminate the most common errors associated with waxing. I suggest that you make a checklist of the waxing techniques and helpful hints mentioned in this chapter and use them as a guide. Practice with friends, family, and clients who are willing to evaluate your work.

Proper Waxing Temperature

The proper temperature for wax application varies with the waxing style of each esthetician. To find your best working temperature, follow these suggestions.

The temperature gauge setting on a wax heater should be set between 60 and 75 degrees centigrade. This temperature seems to produce the consistency of wax needed for a good wax application. If your wax heater has low, medium, and high settings, then the average setting is between medium and high. One of the best ways to tell if wax is of a good consistency and proper temperature is to look at the flow. Dip your spatula in the wax and watch it run off the stick. If the consistency and the flow of wax is like that of honey, it is too cold. If the consistency and flow is more watery, it is too hot. If the flow is more like the flow of syrup (not too thick and not too thin), it's probably just right.

Once you have the consistency that looks just right, test the wax on yourself for heat. You don't have to test the wax on yourself every time. The combination of all three tests—the heater gauge, the flow of wax, and the feel of the wax temperature—will help you recognize the most acceptable temperature by sight. Once you find a good average temperature, keep your wax gauge at this setting; then adjust the temperature up or down as needed. Remember, every client's tolerance will be different, so get in the habit of asking your client if the wax temperature is comfortable. Adjust the wax temperature according to the client's response.

If the client feels that the wax is too hot, lower the temperature gauge. Because of the timing of appointments, you can't wait until the pot of wax is cooled. To cool the wax before applying to the client's skin, blow on it gently.

Before You Apply the Wax

Before you apply wax, you will need to know where you are going to place the wax. Often the epilator will go for the wax, then turn around to see where to pour it; the opposite should be true. Before you wax, stop and think! Ask yourself these questions:

1. What is my objective, and what is the best way for me to perform the service?
2. Did I prepare the area for the wax application?
3. Do I have the proper size muslin for the job?
4. Did I size up the area to be waxed?
5. Did I find out what the client wants?
6. Where am I going to apply the wax first?

An Important Before-You-Wax Fact

If the client's hair is too long, it must be trimmed! What is too long? The hair is too long when it grows beyond the first bend or curve (Figure 4–1). You want the hair to be just long enough to lie flat, approximately $1/4$ inch.

If the hair can't lie flat when the wax is applied, it's too short (Figure 4-2). The proper length is when the hair grows out and begins to curve $1/4$ inch (Figure 4-3). You will have problems if the client's hair is too long and you fail to trim it. First, you can't properly see in which direction the hair is growing. If it's too long, you won't be able to see what direction to apply the wax and what direction to remove the cloth. Second, untrimmed hair results in improper and repeated attempts to remove the hair; you cannot see the direc-

FIGURE 4–1
Hair is too long when it grows beyond the first curve.

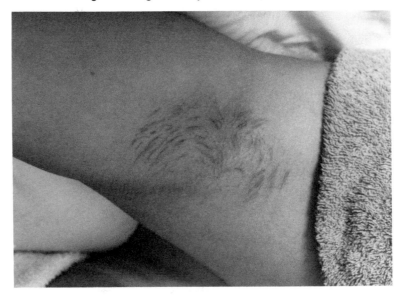

FIGURE 4-2
If the hair won't lie flat when wax is applied, it's too short.

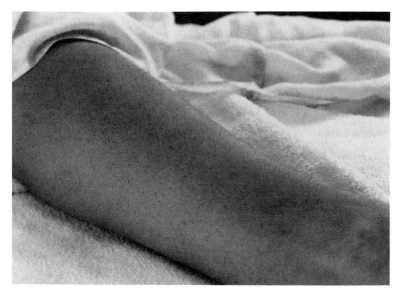

FIGURE 4-3
Proper length is $1/4$ inch.

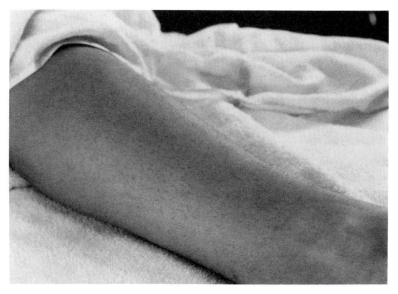

tion of growth. Third, the longer the hair, the more discomfort to the client. Fourth, the longer the hair, the more effort is needed to remove the hair from the shaft. This effort could cause bleeding and bruising. You must trim the hair if it is too long before you wax. Please take your time and trim the hair carefully!

Controlling the Wax

In order to prevent the wax from becoming messy and creating unnecessary problems, you must learn to control it. The best way to control the wax is to remember that it can go only where you direct it. When you take the wax from the heater with the spatula, watch the wax. Hold the wax spatula level from the heater to the area to be waxed. As long as the spatula is level, the wax will not drip or spill (Figures 4-4, 4-5, 4-6). The

FIGURE 4-4
When the spatula is not held level, it will drip or spill.

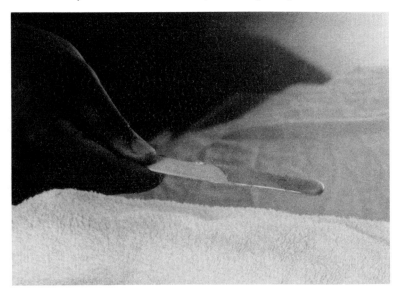

FIGURE 4–5

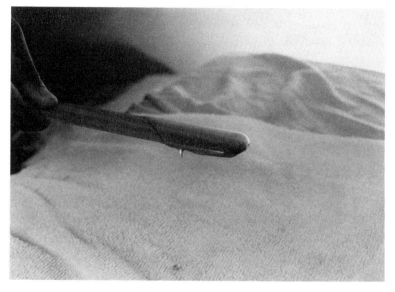

FIGURE 4–6

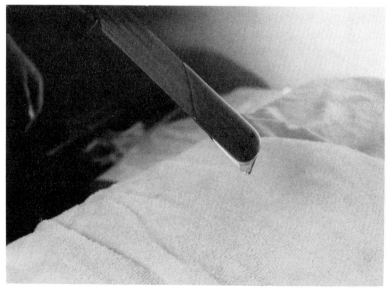

hand position required to wax an area is the same hand position used to take the wax from the heater. There is no room to switch the hand position without some type of spill. If you are waxing an area of the face, you only need a small amount of wax on the top of the spatula (Figure 4–7). If you are waxing the underarms or the bikini line, you need enough wax to cover half of the spatula (Figure 4–8). If you are waxing the legs or the back, you will need enough wax to cover three-quarters of the spatula (Figure 4–9). Start by using a small amount of wax until you build your confidence.

FIGURE 4–7
For the face, only a small amount is needed on the tip of the spatula.

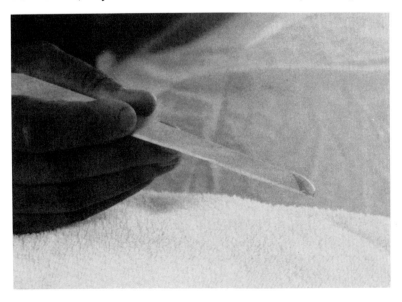

FIGURE 4-8

For the bikini area, wax should cover half of the spatula.

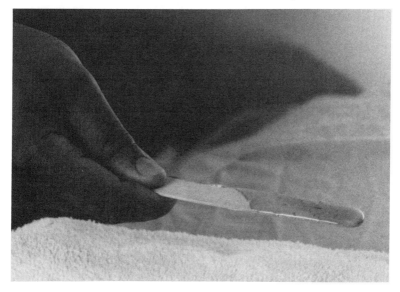

FIGURE 4-9

For the legs, enough wax to cover three-quarters of the spatula is needed.

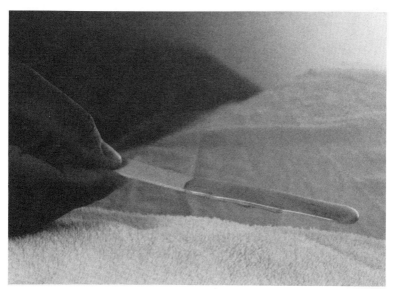

Wax Application

The following is a basic waxing concept. Naturally, there will be exceptions. We will later discuss individual requirements for specific areas (Chapter 7).

The rule for waxing is as follows: Apply the wax in the direction of the hair growth. The wax application should be smooth, thin, and even. Apply muslin over the applied wax, leaving 1 to 2 inches of free cloth (Figure 4–10) for gripping. Smooth the cloth into place with two to three light strokes (Figure 4–11). Hold the skin taut with the opposite hand, and pull the cloth quickly in the opposite direction of the hair growth (Figure 4–12). Tap quickly and lightly over the waxed area. As simple as it may sound, it can be com-

FIGURE 4–10
Leave 1 to 2 inches of free cloth for gripping.

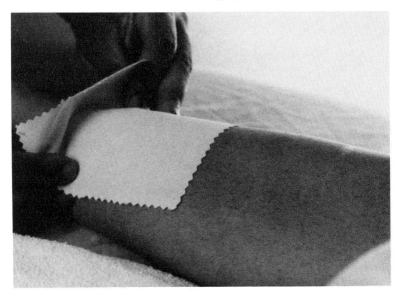

FIGURE 4–11
Smooth cloth into place with two or three light strokes.

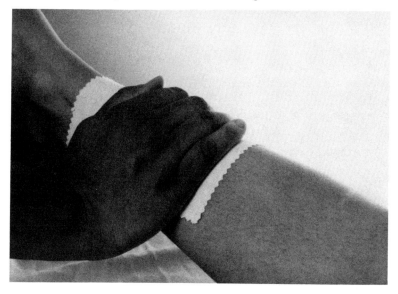

FIGURE 4–12
Hold skin taut while pulling in the opposite direction of hair growth.

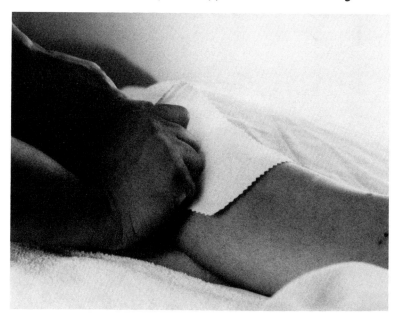

plicated if certain techniques are not employed. Follow these few techniques:

Technique #1: Wax Application

Hold the spatula so you won't have to change position once the spatula reaches the area to be waxed. Hold the spatula at a 45 degree angle (Figure 4–13). At a 45 degree angle, you can see the wax as it is being applied. If your wax stick is at less than a 45 degree angle, you won't be able to see the wax being applied. If your wax stick is at less than a 30 degree angle, you will prevent the flow of wax (Figure 4–14). At a 30 degree angle, your wax won't go very far. The wax will be applied thickly and unevenly. One way to practice this technique is to put an inexpensive cold cream on the spatula. Find a large piece of cardboard; take your spatula with the cream and, starting from the top of the

FIGURE 4–13
Hold spatula at a 45 degree angle during wax application.

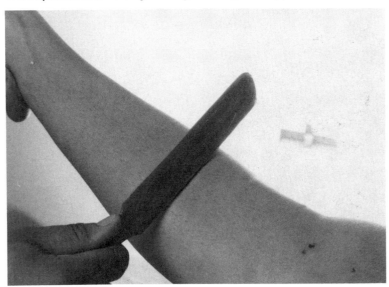

FIGURE 4-14
If the spatula is at a 30 degree angle or less, you'll be unable to see the application.

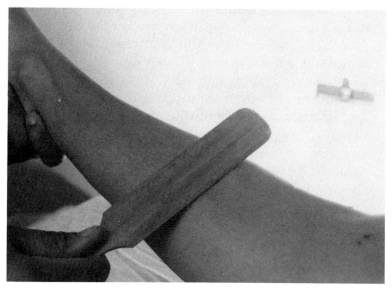

cardboard, hold your stick at a 45 degree angle and spread downward, making several strokes side by side. Look at your cream application. Was the cold cream applied evenly, smoothly, and thinly? Did you scrape the board with the spatula? If the spatula scrapes the board, the cream will not flow well. The same is true for waxing. In order for the wax to flow evenly, the spatula should barely touch the skin. Practice this sequence until you feel you have mastered holding the spatula at a constant 45 degree angle. Practice until the cream is applied evenly and smoothly. Practice until the strokes become natural.

Technique #2: Removal of the Wax

Removal of the wax is just as important as the application. The type and size of the cloth affect the ease of removing the wax. (Chapter 2). Once the wax is applied, a properly cut muslin strip is applied over the wax, allowing 1 $^1/_2$ to 2 inches for a free edge for gripping. Smooth the cloth with the palm of the hand (do not pat, press, or use fingers) in the direction of hair growth. This adheres the cloth to the wax and the hair follicles. It is not necessary to apply much pressure or to rub the cloth more than twice. If you rub the cloth until the wax bleeds through, you may cause unnecessary irritation to the client when removing. With the opposite hand, pull the skin taut in the same direction as the hair growth. Hold that taut position firmly. Grip the free edge of the cloth firmly with the waxing hand. Quickly, pull the cloth in the opposite direction of the hair growth, keeping the hand close to the skin. Release the opposite hand and use it now to tap quickly over the waxed area. (Review this sequence several times.)

Technique #3: The Position of the Cloth

One way to tell if you are on the right track is to observe your cloth during and after a waxing session. Keep these techniques in mind:

1. Keep the cloth close to the area being waxed during removal.

2. Tell yourself to hold the skin taut with one hand, with the other pull the cloth back quickly, and keep the hand close to the skin (Figure 4–15).

3. Stop your hand once you have pulled the cloth away (Figure 4–16). Do not let your hand go in any direction (up in the air, over your head, etc.) (Figure 4–17).

4. After waxing, look at your hand. Is it in the air or close to the area being waxed? (Figure 4–18.) Is it straight ahead of you? Are you tapping with your other hand?

FIGURE 4–15
Pull skin taut with one hand; pull the cloth with the other.

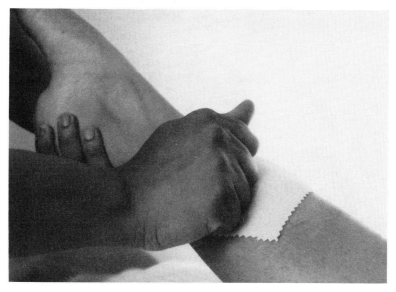

FIGURE 4–16
Stop your hand once you have pulled the cloth away.

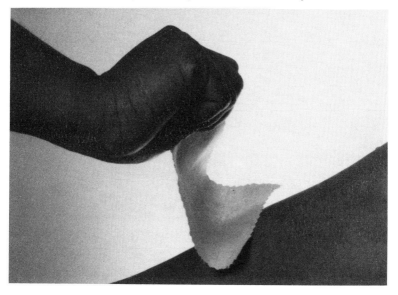

FIGURE 4–17
Cloth should not be held up in the air or in any other direction.

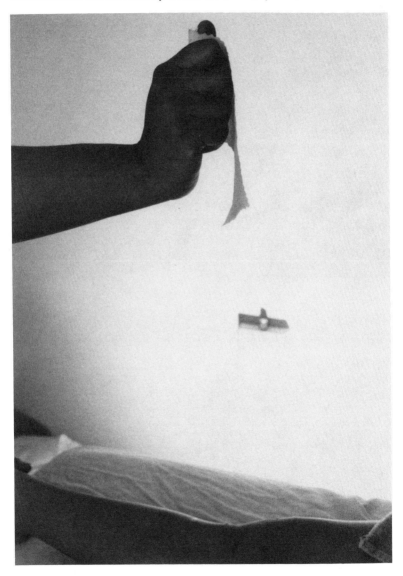

FIGURE 4-18
Cloth should be close to the area being waxed.

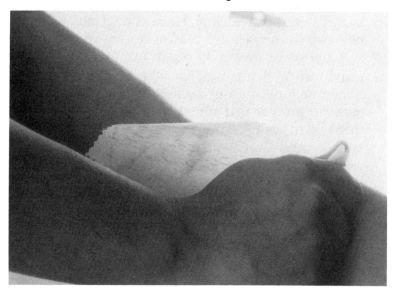

Technique #4: Tapping and Slapping

Tapping and slapping are very beneficial to the client. After you remove the wax, give a light tapping (small area) and slapping (large area). Tapping lessens the discomfort you feel from the hair being pulled from the hair shaft. Tapping and slapping confuses the signal the brain is receiving. Once the cloth is removed, the nerve endings register pain; then when you are being tapped or slapped the brain receives a new, added sensation. The new sensation is that of pressure. The signal of pain is now lessened. Immediately after you snatch a removal cloth from the skin, start tapping and slapping.

Technique #5: Holding the Skin Taut

The structure of the hair follicle includes a muscle attached to the hair follicle and sebaceous glands. We do not want to contract that muscle because contracting it would stimulate the oil gland. Stimulating the oil gland will fill the hair follicle with an abundance of unnecessary oil, causing bumping. Holding the skin taut will prevent that stimulation. Remember, every inch of skin has 1,300 nerve endings. Holding the skin taut prevents overstimulation of the nerve endings and lessens the discomfort the client feels. Also, the skin is very elastic, and if it is not held taut, the skin will give with the pull of muslin and snap back so abruptly that it will bruise.

Review of Basic Techniques

Below is a list of some depilatory waxing techniques and helpful hints:

1. Keep yourself and your wax area free of wax spills. Keep your wax stick level when carrying wax.

2. Always lay your wax stick across the top of the heater and not on a table.

3. Wax with your hand close to the skin, never snatching the muslin upward.

4. Muslin strips can be used up to three or four times before disposing (exceptions are the brow and lip).

5. When using the wax strips again, hold the free edge with one hand and grip opposite end corner with your fingers. Where there is little or no wax, apply.

6. Use talcum powder before waxing to absorb oil and perspiration.

7. Keep all waxing instruments clean and free of wax during the procedure. Take the time to dispose or clean wax residue left on the spatulas.

8. To remove the wax residue on the skin, reapply the muslin cloth, smooth as normal, and remove as normal.

9. Do not ball the cloth and tap it over the wax residue when trying to remove it. Popping the cloth and tapping over the wax residue is very uncomfortable.

10. Place a towel over the client's clothing for protection.

11. Do not reapply wax over an area where hair has been removed (Chapter 9).

12. Wearing rubber gloves is a personal choice; however, if you or the client have an open cut, you should wear gloves.

13. Petroleum jelly and heavy oils are good for cleaning equipment, but not for removing residue from the skin (Chapter 8).

14. Removing the muslin should make a certain sound. It is a steady, even, swish sound. The sound should not be harsh, as in ripping. Learn to listen for a good, steady swish!

15. When you grip the muslin to remove wax, do not lift the cloth too high. You may lift the muslin from the wax and leave the hair covered with the wax (a common mistake in brow and lip waxing).

16. When waxing, plant feet firmly on the ground; the back is straight. All areas should be reached without bending or excessive stretching. The only moving parts during waxing should be your hands, wrists, arms, and shoulders.

17. Apply wax in the direction of the hair growth; pull the muslin cloth in the opposite direction.

18. Tweeze one or two hairs only. The client came for a waxing, not a tweezing.

19. Concentrate, and learn to be a perfectionist!

20. When removing the wax, remember, the quicker the better.

This chapter contains a lot of essential information for the epilator. I suggest that you read the material several times. Review the techniques and the helpful hints. Make a checklist to see if you have forgotten techniques. When practicing, talk out loud when applicable. When reviewing the steps, go through the motions several times.

Now that you understand the basic concept of waxing, let's learn how to wax specific areas.

REVIEW QUESTIONS

1. What are the five basic waxing steps?

2. How should the temperature of the wax be tested?

3. What step should be done before the waxing begins?

4. What five points should be considered when starting the waxing procedure?

5. Why is it important to control the wax?

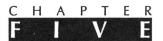

C H A P T E R
F I V E

Let's Wax

CHAPTER OBJECTIVES

1. To discuss in detail the various steps in waxing

2. To lead the epilator through the different steps of waxing various areas of the body, including brows, chin, lower legs, upper thighs, arms, underarms, the bikini area, the back, and the face

When you read "proceed with the wax process," use the techniques discussed in Chapter 4. You should understand and be able to use the standard waxing procedure before going on to these individual steps.

If this is the client's first time experiencing hair removal you will want to explain the procedure. Let the client know that there can be some discomfort. Explain the possible sensations. Tell your client about the possibility of redness and some slight swelling. Your client should also know that these conditions are temporary and should not last for more than twenty minutes.

It is important to remember that the facial areas have an abundance of sebaceous glands. An epilator can overstimulate the sebaceous glands by waxing too large an area at one time. The long, excessive pulling will cause white pustules to surface. Therefore, it is best to take smaller strips, approximately $1\frac{1}{2}$ to 2 inches wide by 4 to 5 inches long for small areas and adjust your strips to the size of the area being waxed. This chapter will recommend cloth sizes.

You can begin waxing procedures from two positions. One of those positions is behind the esthetic chair. The other position is facing the client. Generally, when waxing the brows, lips, and chin, the proper position is to stand behind the client (Figure 5–1) with the chair at a 60 degree angle. If you do not have a chair that can lean backwards, you should stand next to your client, while facing the client. Now that we have everything in place (materials, good sanitation procedures, and a good attitude), I want to share with you a personal goal: not to tweeze more than 5 hairs during any waxing session (the exception here would be the technique for hair stubble mentioned in Chapter 7). If you take this as your goal too you will want to move with accurate and precise steps. Let's wax!

Brows

Measure the proper brow shape for client. Align a pencil along the inside corner of the eye (Figure 5–2); all hair outside the pencil should be waxed. Now place the pencil outside the iris of the eye (Figure 5–3); this is were the arch should begin. Last, place the pencil at an angle from the side of the client's nose to the outside corner of the eye (Figure 5–4). This is where the brow tapers and ends. I would advise a discussion with the client concerning her desired brow shape before waxing.

Take a small amount of wax on the tip of the spatula designed for waxing brows; wipe the back of the spatula clean; lift the brow with your free hand; and begin to apply the wax over the hairs that you want to remove. Your stroke should be smooth and continuous.

FIGURE 5-1

Stand behind the client with the chair at a 60 degree angle.

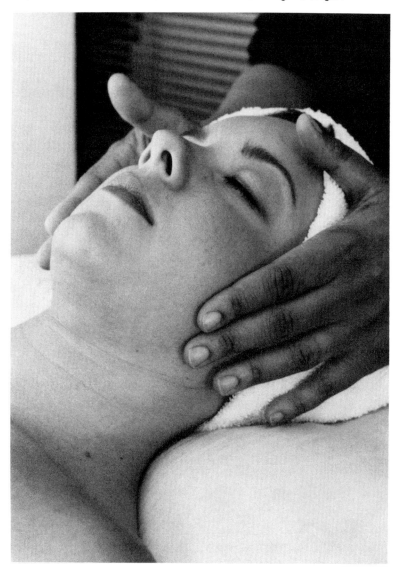

FIGURE 5-2

For the start of the brow, align the pencil along the inside corner of the eye.

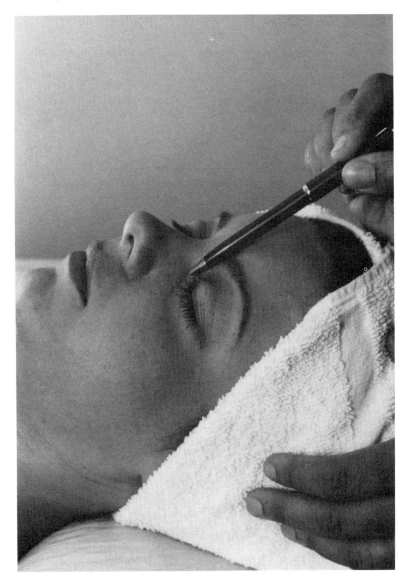

FIGURE 5–3
For the arch of the brow, place the pencil on the outside of the iris of the eye.

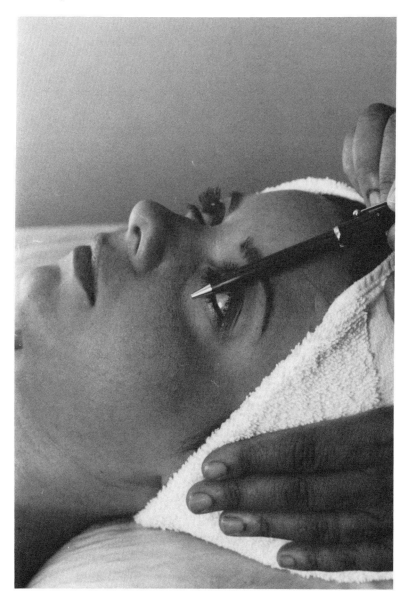

FIGURE 5–4
For the end of the brow, place the pencil at an angle along the side
of the nose to the outside corner of the eye.

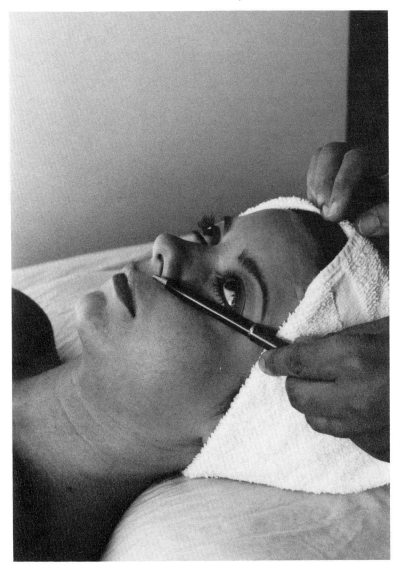

Be careful not to drip wax from the spatula onto hairs you want to keep. Be sure to hold the spatula away from hairs you do not want to wax (Figure 5-5). Take your time! Now carefully pull the waxed hairs down and away from the brow (Figure 5-6). You should be able to see the shape of the brow (Figure 5-7). You should also be able to see if you have any hairs that should be removed, but are not covered with wax. If you do see where your brow is not properly shaped, and you want to remove more hair, then with the very edge of your spatula pull the undesired hairs into the applied wax. Before you apply the muslin strip assess your work. Are you pleased with the wax application? Is there any wax where you don't want it? (If so, then be sure not to place a muslin strip over that part of the brow.) Now take your muslin strip and place over the wax. Make sure to leave a free edge for grasping. Smooth the muslin strip with light pressure. You should be able to see the wax under the strip. Grasp the free edge of the strip firmly between your index finger and thumb. (Figure 5-8). Hold the skin taut on the outside of the corner of the eye with your other hand. Now, while you have your strip grasped firmly and the skin pulled taut, pull your strip quickly in the opposite direction of hair growth (Figure 5-9), keeping the hand close to the skin (Figure 5-10). (Refer to Chapter 4 for waxing techniques.) Tap the skin with your opposite finger quickly. Discard the muslin strip. If there are one or two hairs that you did not remove, then tweeze them. If there are quite a few hairs left, then you must reapply the wax only over the hairs that you want to remove! You must not reapply wax to any area where you have already removed hair! If you were to apply wax on a area where the hair has been removed you would cause a burn. Take a very small amount of wax and apply it to the hairs only; follow through with the muslin strip and the hair removal technique. Look at

FIGURE 5-5
Hold the spatula away from hairs not to be waxed.

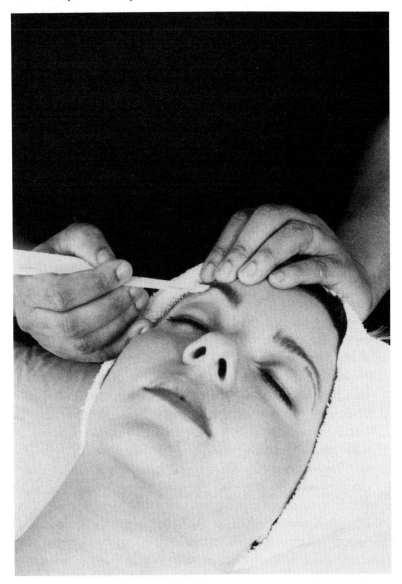

FIGURE 5–6
Pull the waxed hairs down and away from the brow.

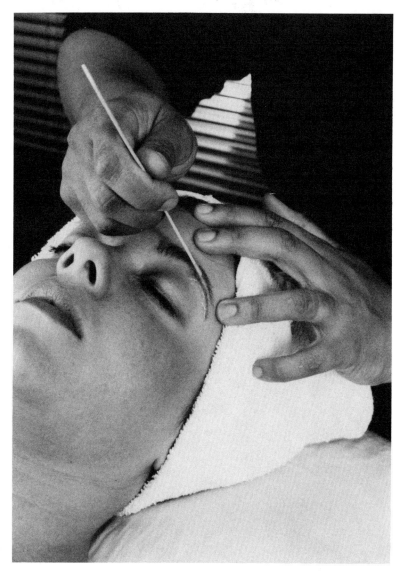

FIGURE 5–7
You should be able to see the shape of the brow.

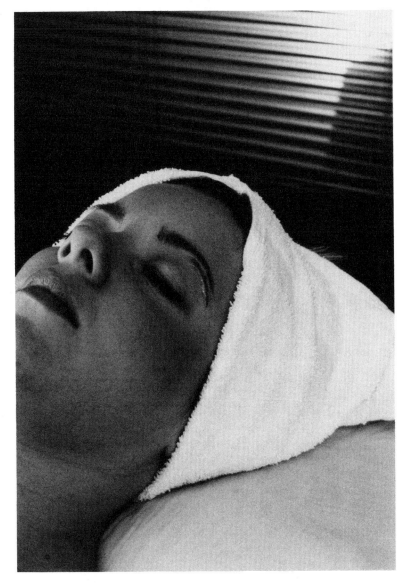

FIGURE 5-8
Grasp the free edge of the strip between the index finger and thumb.

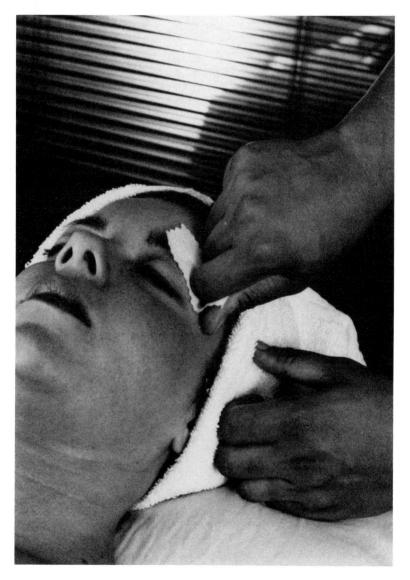

FIGURE 5–9
Hold skin taut; pull the strip in the opposite direction of hair growth.

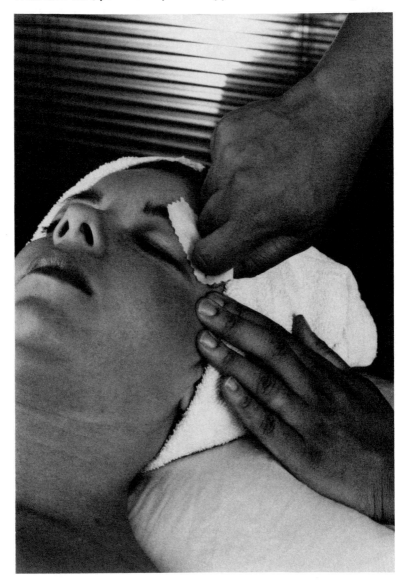

FIGURE 5–10
Keep your hand close to the skin.

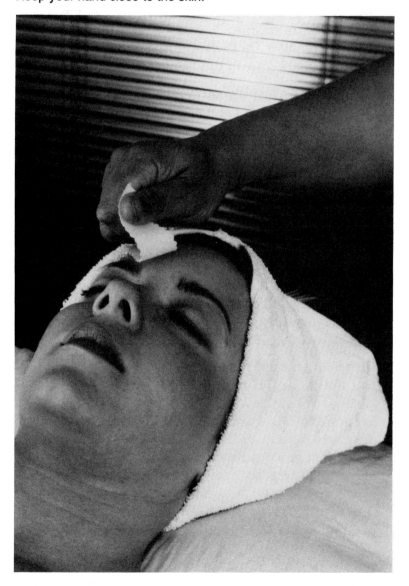

your work, and if you are pleased, apply the proper protection cream (Figure 5–11). Note: some epilators like to apply powder (talc, cornstarch, or a commercial brand) before waxing. This step ensures that all oils and perspiration are absorbed. You should use your own personal choice in this manner.

One way to develop a good eye for shaping brows is to measure the brows for proper shape, then draw on that shape with an eyebrow pencil and wax all other hairs.

Before removing hair from the top of the brows and along the hairline, you should always discuss it with the client.

Above the Lip

Understanding the direction in which the hair grows above the upper lip will help you understand this waxing technique. To avoid small bumping and skin irritation, wax the hair in four sections.

Hair above the upper lip generally grows in four different directions (Figure 5-12). The first section is the side of the lip; that hair grows downward. The second section generally grows at a slight angle. Each area will be waxed separately. Starting with the outside corners, apply wax in a downward stroke, being sure to cover all the hair (especially in the corners of the mouth). Apply your muslin strip, and smooth it until you see the wax under the cloth. Grasp the muslin between the thumb and forefinger (Figure 5-13). Hold the skin taut with the other hand; now quickly remove the muslin, pulling in the opposite direction of the hair growth. Tap the skin quickly. Repeat the procedure on the other corner. When waxing the middle portion of the lip, divide the lip into two sections. Wax one section at a time. First apply the wax in a downward di-

FIGURE 5–11
Apply proper protection cream.

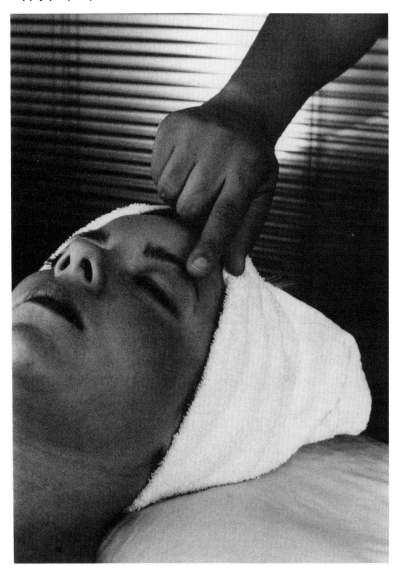

FIGURE 5–12
Hair on the upper lip grows in different directions.

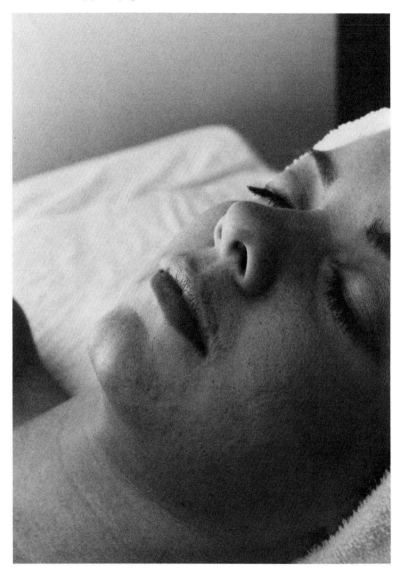

FIGURE 5–13
Grasp muslin between the thumb and forefinger.

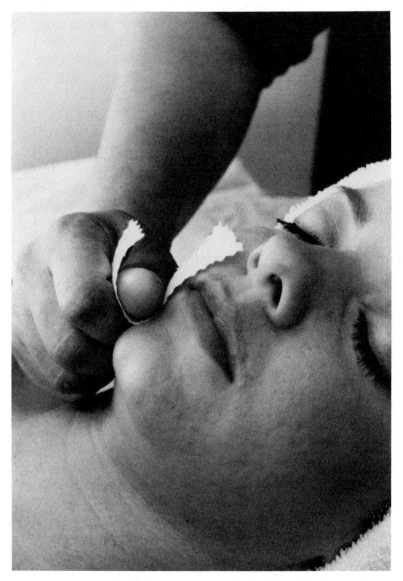

rection over the top of the lip, covering all the hair (apply over the edge of the lip to cover minute, fine hairs). Proceed with the wax procedure. Apply the muslin strip at an angle, leaving a free edge to grasp (Figure 5–14). Have the client curve her lip over her teeth, to make the top lip taut. The reason we apply the cloth at an angle is to avoid interference with the nose, and because most hair grows at an angle. Grasp the muslin cloth between the thumb and forefinger. Quickly remove the cloth in the opposite direction of the hair growth. Tap the area quickly. Repeat the process with the other section. Apply the proper afterlotion. I find the above technique to be more effective than waxing the upper lip in two movements. It puts less stress on pulling the muslin, and with less stress on the lip area there is less chance of fine pustules forming. The client experiences less discomfort.

The Chin

Waxing the chin can be the easiest of all the facial waxing areas. Normally all hairs grow in the same direction. Holding the skin taut is easier. You should begin at the base of the chin. Use small strips, approximately $1\,^1/_2$ by 4 inches. Remember when applying the muslin strip to leave enough space to grasp the muslin strip. Cover the entire base of the chin with wax. Apply the muslin strip over a portion of the wax, and smooth the muslin until the wax shows through. Holding the skin taut with the other hand, pull the muslin cloth in the opposite direction of hair growth (Figure 5–15). Apply the same muslin strip over your next wax section. Repeat the waxing procedure. Move to your next section and repeat the process. The base area being waxed should not require more than three or four strips to remove the hair. If your client requires

FIGURE 5–14

Apply the muslin strip at an angle, leaving a free edge to grasp.

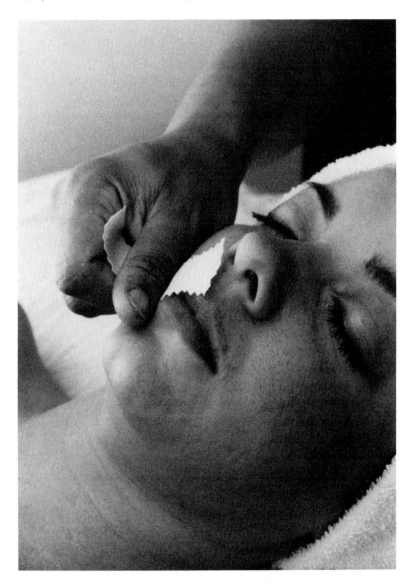

FIGURE 5–15
Hold skin taut on the chin and pull in the opposite direction of hair growth.

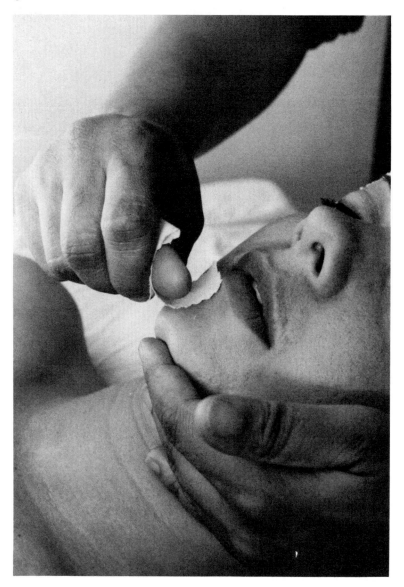

more than three pulls, then I suggest that you change the muslin strip after three pulls. If the wax is applied smoothly and thinly, you can generally use the muslin strips for three or four pulls before disposing. We now want to move up to the next section of the chin. Repeat the process that you used for the base of the chin. Once you have finished the chin area apply the proper afterlotion. If you run into short stubble refer to Chapter 7, which covers that problem. Sometimes the client's chin includes the neck area (Figure 5–16). If that is the case, divide the chin and the neck areas into three sections. By dividing the chin into three sections you can eliminate discomfort and fine pustules.

Lower Legs

I would advise any beginner to begin practicing waxing on the legs. The area is large enough to develop good application and stroke techniques, and, generally, the hairs all grow in one direction. Prepare the area to be waxed. Have waxing strips approximately 4 by 9 $1/2$ inches. Apply wax to an area of 3 by 7 inches to begin (Figure 5–17). After you have learned control and a good pulling stroke the need to measure will be eliminated. Apply the muslin cloth over the area, leaving a free edge. Smooth the cloth until you see the wax bleed through. Grasp the free edge with your thumb and forefinger (Figure 5–18). Hold the skin taut with your opposite hand. Pull the muslin cloth straight back in the opposite direction of hair growth. Tap the area quickly to ease any discomfort (Figure 5–19). Move to the next section and repeat the procedure. I suggest that you start at the ankles and move right to left. Move upward to the next section until you reach the knee. Once you have waxed the front of the legs have your client turn over so you can repeat the pro-

FIGURE 5–16
Sometimes the client's chin includes the neck area.

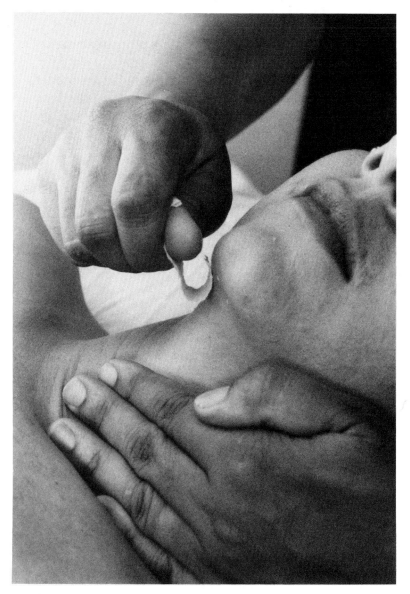

FIGURE 5–17
Cover an area 3 by 7 inches with wax.

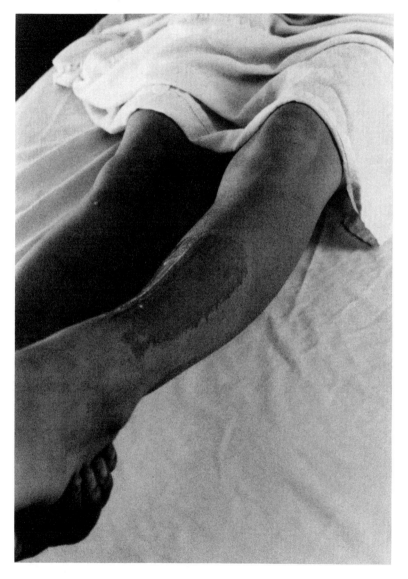

FIGURE 5–18
Grasp the free edge with the thumb and forefinger.

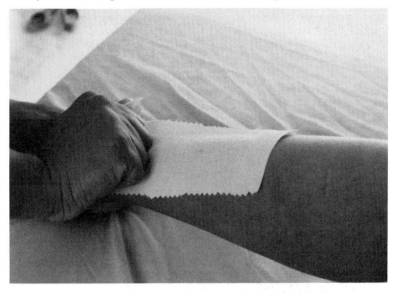

FIGURE 5–19
Tap area quickly to ease discomfort.

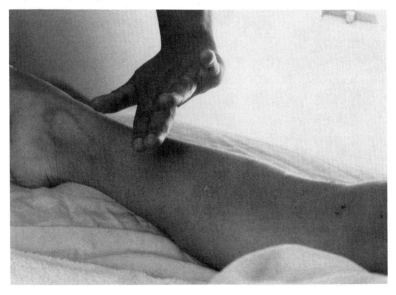

cedure on the back of the legs. Some epilators like to wax the knees before turning the client over. With this in mind let's wax the knees. You must have the client bend the knees (Figure 5-20). This will keep the knee smooth and taut. Divide the knee in two sections, top to bottom. Apply wax to the bottom half of the knee. Use smaller strips (approximately half the size of the leg strip). Follow the wax procedure. Follow the same procedure for the top knee. When waxing the knee, be sure to include the sides of the knee. For the top part of the knee, hold the knee taut at the lower thigh. After removing each strip be sure to apply the tapping technique to ease discomfort.

Upper Thigh

Waxing the upper thigh is a lot different than the lower leg. The hair on the upper thigh grows in different directions. You have to wax each section in a different direction. I suggest you begin with the top of the leg, then wax the inside of the thigh, and proceed to the outside side of the thigh. Repeat this pattern on the front of the other thigh. Once you have completed both thighs turn the client over and wax the back of the thighs. You will find the hair on the back of the legs growing in one direction. Use the same technique as you used for the lower leg. The area for waxing the upper leg ends at the panty brief line. When waxing the upper thigh you have to be sure to hold the thigh extremely taut. The thigh will bruise very easily, because the skin is more flaccid than that of the leg. To ensure that the leg is taut have your client help you. Have your client hold the thigh by grasping it underneath and pulling back the flesh. You can hold the skin taut when it comes to removing the muslin strip.

FIGURE 5–20
Have the client bend the knee.

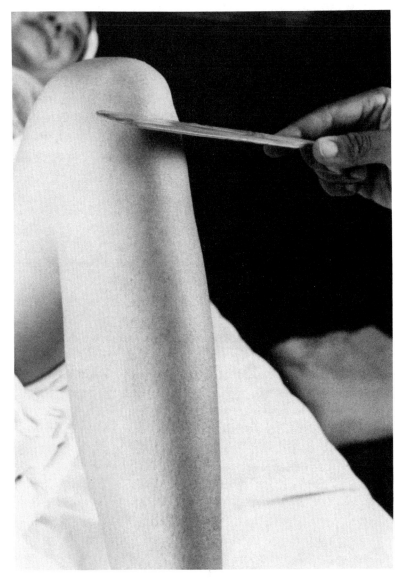

Arms

Many women would like to have their arms waxed because of excessive or dark hair. The hair on the arm grows in different directions. If too large strips are used, large bumps may appear. The best strip size for waxing arms is 3 by 6 inches. Begin waxing the arms on top. The hair on top of the arms usually grows sideways. Hold the client's hand and extend the arm until it is comfortable for you to apply the wax. Do not go beyond the elbow at this point. Bend the arm up and apply wax on any downward hairs. The client can be a support here. Remember you must still hold the skin taut. Now have the client bend the arm so the elbow is pointing out. Take smaller strips that are designed for brows or chins and wax the elbow. You can now proceed to the upper arms if the client desires. If the hair on the arms is long, take the time to clip it down. This will eliminate overstimulation of the sebaceous glands and discomfort. Remember your waxing techniques and tips.

Underarms

Waxing the underarms is a common practice for women. Epilators should tell clients about this service because of its convenience and the length of time before having to repeat the service. The ideal candidate is a person whose hair growth is not coarse. Medium to fine hair is more likely to respond to the four to six weeks' regrowth pattern. Have your client place her lower arm in back of her head (Figure 5–21). This position will stretch the armpits. You may want at this point to check the length of hair. If it is too long, then you want to clip the hair. Apply powder to this area to absorb excessive moisture. You will notice that the hair grows in several directions (Figure 5–22); each

FIGURE 5–21

Have the client place her lower arm behind her head.

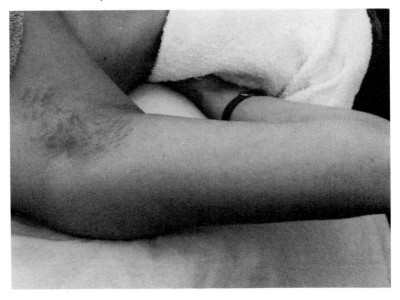

FIGURE 5–22

Underarm hair grows in several directions.

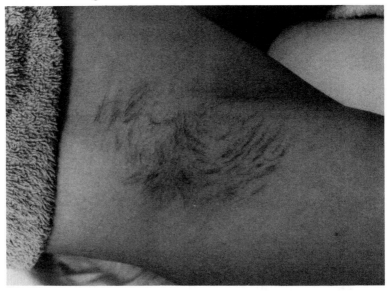

section must be waxed separately. Since each area being waxed is small, apply a small amount of wax to each section (Figure 5-23). Be sure to hold the skin taut when waxing each section (Figure 5-24). Occasionally some stubble will be noticed after waxing; if so, refer to Chapter 7 on removing hair stubble and follow that procedure. Some tips on waxing underarms: clean the area with a precleaning solution to remove any chemicals on the skin. Remove the largest patches of hair first. Remove all the hair; it would defeat the purpose of coming if the client has to go home and shave any portion of hair. Use an antiseptic after waxing, because this will help eliminate the possibility of cysts. (Some clients are prone to cysts in the underarms due to ingrown hairs deep in the skin.) Advise the client not to use underarm protection until the next day. You should powder the arms well after the after-lotion has been applied.

Bikini Line

Besides the brow and lip, bikini line waxing is the next most popular waxing procedure. The preparation for bikini waxing should be as follows: Have the client remove underwear and place between the legs a clean towel or put on disposable underwear (Figure 5-25). I suggest this practice because sanitation is strongly encouraged today. The towel can be manipulated so you never have to touch it. Today's bathing suit designs are cut in various styles. Your client can adjust the towel to expose the hair she wants removed. Underwear is not designed for waxing, so the epilator might have to touch a client's underwear to reach the hair to be removed. After the procedure you can sanitize the towel with bleach when cleaning. The disposable un-

FIGURE 5–23
Apply a small amount of wax to each section.

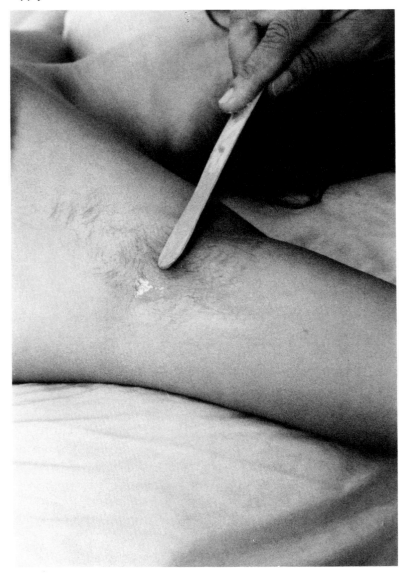

FIGURE 5–24
Be sure to hold skin taut when waxing each section.

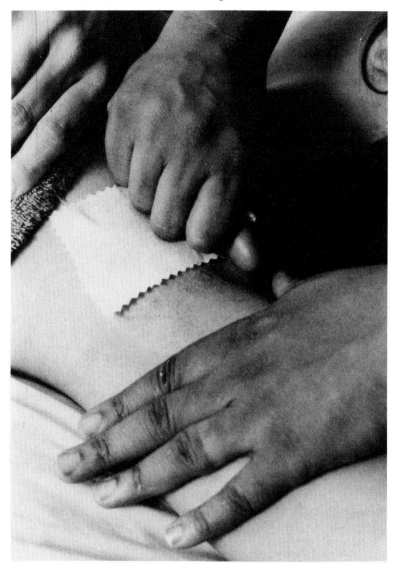

FIGURE 5–25
Have the client place a clean towel between the legs.

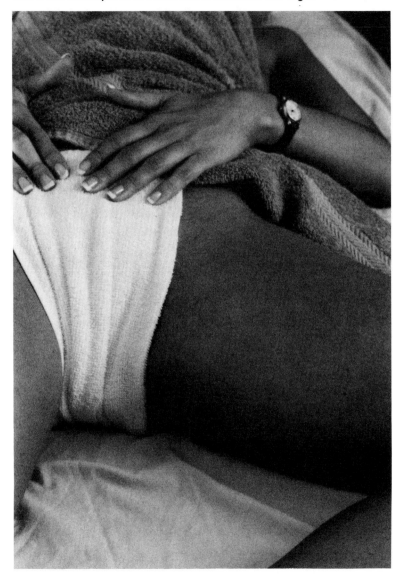

derwear can be discarded; however, they are expensive.

You should always trim the hair if it is too long. Precleaning the area is advised. Powder is suggested to absorb moisture.

Position the client with the leg raised so the bikini area is exposed and the thigh lies flat on the table (Figure 5–26). Your client can assist you by reaching under the leg and holding the flesh taut. Once you have become more skilled you probably will be able to eliminate this procedure. Apply wax over any hairs on the top of the thigh first. Proceed with the waxing process. Be sure to hold the skin taut. Your waxing strips should be 3 by 6 inches. Move up to your next section (the pelvic area). Apply wax in the direction of growth. When pulling the strip from this area you may want to hold the skin on the thigh close to the area to be waxed. When waxing the inside of the pelvic area (Figure 5–27), you must be sure the hair is trimmed and you must remember to hold the skin very taut. This area is a common place for bruising to occur. Apply a small amount of wax. Proceed with the waxing process. Hair growing close to the buttocks may require the client to bend her knee (Figure 5–28). Apply the wax in the direction of the hair growth and remove the muslin cloth in the opposite direction. Remember these basic points when waxing the bikini area: (1) Use a small amount of wax. (2) Trim the hair. (3) Hold the skin taut and close to the area being waxed. (4) Divide the bikini line into three or four sections for control. (5) After the procedure, apply an antiseptic and powder. If a client complains of any discomfort or a small irritation, suggest a baking soda and water bath (one box to a tub of water). (6) Advise clients not to expose themselves to the sun for twenty-four hours.

FIGURE 5–26
Raise the leg so the bikini area is exposed and the thigh is lying flat on the table.

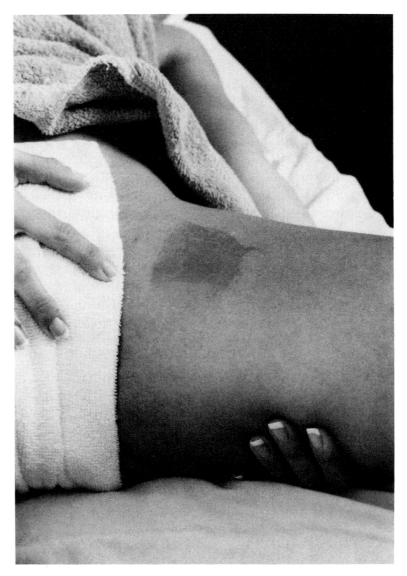

FIGURE 5-27
Make sure the hair is trimmed when waxing inside the pelvic area.

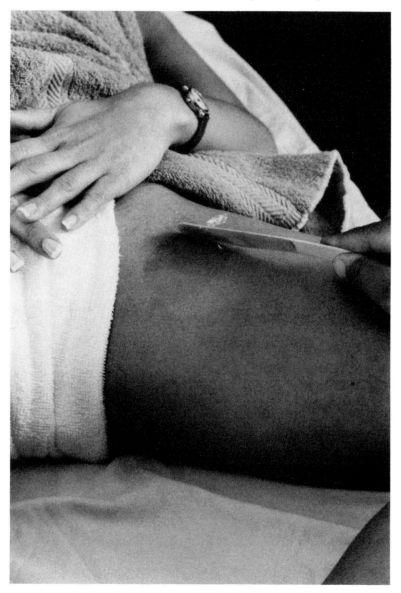

FIGURE 5–28
Hair growing close to the buttocks may require the client to bend the knee.

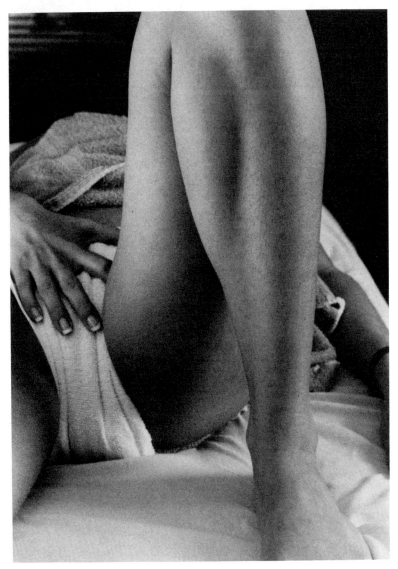

Backs

Male clients will often request that hair be removed from the back area. This procedure can be an uncomfortable process for the client. To ensure good results, follow these tips. Trim all the hair. Follow a pattern starting at the back of the neckline and completing the procedure at the waist. Your waxing strips should be no longer than 3 by 8 inches. Trying to wax a large area of the back at one time will result in pustules. Once you have completed the waxing procedure apply an ice cold compress of baking soda and water (one tablespoon of baking soda to a pint of water to which ice cubes have been added). The back will become stimulated, and you can tell this by the amount of heat generated. The cold compress should not last longer than fifteen minutes. Wipe the back clean with a damp cloth. Apply antiseptic cream.

Face

Waxing the face is a procedure desired mostly by women. We can remove soft facial hair by depilatory waxing. The procedure does require time and patience. A small amount of wax should be applied in a thin layer. The size of the strips should not exceed 1 $\frac{1}{2}$ by 4 inches. You must establish a pattern. The best way is to begin with the chin, proceed to the left and right cheeks, and then work your way up to the forehead. Stick with your pattern so you won't miss any hairs. The preparation for waxing the face is the same as for all waxing. Encourage your client to come with her makeup removed. Makeup will cause overstimulation and the application of an oil base product for removal. She must understand that to get the best results you should manipulate the skin as little as possible. Waxing the face alone can cause overstimulation of the sebaceous glands. It is very common for clients to experience small pustules. Holding the skin taut is very important, and a gentle touch is necessary. Once you have completed the waxing procedure you must apply the baking soda and water compress. Be sure to use ice in the water; it will cool the face. The baking soda and water will promote disincrustation and prevent small pustules. The client should use the antiseptic lotion at home for a day or two. If the client complains of small pustules, inform the client that they are temporary and advise applying baking soda and water to the skin at home for fifteen minutes. This will help dry up the pustule more quickly.

The individual procedures that we just reviewed will help you in waxing. The key point to remember is that if you take your time, you will actually save time. Adjust your strip size to the size of the job being done. Adjust the quantity of the wax to be applied to an area. Other than the leg area, only small amounts of wax are required to remove hair. When it comes to waxing any area on the face only a small amount of wax is needed. Start with a small amount of wax, then add more if needed; if you follow this rule you can save yourself many mistakes. Confidence comes with time, so be patient.

REVIEW QUESTIONS

1. Name three important factors to keep in mind when waxing the brows, lips, bikini area, and facial hair.

2. What is the goal of the waxing procedure?

3. After waxing a client's back, what steps are taken to ease discomfort?

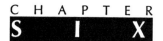

Aftercare

CHAPTER OBJECTIVES

1. To learn how to properly treat the client after a waxing procedure
2. To inform the epilator of alternatives to after-waxing care

There is a general after-waxing care procedure that is standard; however, certain areas require specific care. We will discuss both of these.

General care includes checking the area being waxed for any residue. If there is any wax residue, place a muslin cloth over the area and follow with the waxing procedure. This will ensure that all residue is removed. Do not pop the cloth over the wax residue. This is uncomfortable for the client, and it does not ensure complete removal. Clean the area with afterwax lotion (antiseptic) and apply the aftercare lotion (protection cream).

Disincrustation

Another aftercare procedure is using baking soda and water. A baking soda and water solution promotes disincrustation. A disincrustation helps to emulsify oils and also serves as a calming solution for most skin rashes and irritations. For areas where sebaceous glands may become overstimulated, apply baking soda solution (1 tablespoon to a pint of water) by means of a cotton compress for twenty minutes. The area that needs it most would be the back, the arms, and the face. When your client informs you of previous bumping in a particular area after waxing add a compress of baking soda and water to the area. Add ice to the baking soda solution to help cool the skin. Sometimes when waxing an area for a long period of time the skin can become warm. The cool solution will help this situation.

High-Frequency Current

High-frequency current is also very good for destroying bacteria and preventing the development of cysts. The areas that would benefit from high-frequency current are the underarms, back, bikini area, and face.

Dr. Jock's Wort Oil is excellent for taking redness out. I would apply it to the brows and lips. This would be a good product to sell in your salon. Application of powder after the aftercare lotion will ease any irritation caused by friction. The areas that would benefit from this application would be the bikini area and the underarms.

You should remember that waxing can cause skin irritations. Most clients will respond positively to waxing. However, a few clients can respond negatively to waxing, so you should practice special aftercare steps to ensure the best response to the service. Certain areas are prone to pustules, papules, and skin sensitivity. You need to be aware of all the possible options for treating the conditions. This awareness will ensure a satisfied client.

REVIEW QUESTIONS

1. How does a solution of baking soda and water help if there is discomfort after waxing?
2. What equipment is used after waxing facial hairs?
3. What should be done after a waxing procedure?
4. What product is used to reduce irritation caused by friction after waxing?

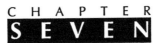

What Do I Do Now?

CHAPTER OBJECTIVES

1. To show the epilator how to properly help a client with pseudofolliculitis

2. To show how to remove hair stubble

3. To discuss solutions to problems that arise during waxing

Sometimes, even when your technique is flawless, you will run into problems. In this chapter we will discuss some of the more common situations and what you should do about them.

Pseudofolliculitis

Pseudofolliculitis is a disorder of the hair follicle—the hair follicle curves back into the skin. This disorder causes several problems. Pustules, skin irritations, and pus can develop. In males shaving complications also occur. To alleviate these complications, you can follow these procedures: (1) Use a sterile lancet to lift the hair that is embedded. Take a blunt edged tweezer, grasp the hair follicle at the base of the hair next to the skin, and pull the hair in the direction of growth. Keep the tweezer close to the skin during this procedure.

Apply a medicated lotion over the affected area. (2) When working with males who have a large number of ingrown hairs, I suggest a facial treatment that will prepare the skin for epilation and smooth the skin after epilation. The procedure is as follows: Cleanse the client's skin. Make a cotton compress of baking soda disincrustation (one tablespoon of baking soda to a pint of water). This will emulsify the oil deposits around the hair follicle. Apply the compress to the affected area. A vaporizer could be used during these fifteen minutes. After removing the compress rinse the skin. With the use of a magnifying lamp (5 Diopter) use a sterilized lancet to lift every hair that is embedded under the skin. With your tweezer grasp the hair follicle and pull the hair in the direction of hair growth. Keep the tweezer close to the skin during this procedure. Once you have removed the curved hair from the follicle apply a medicated mask designed for healing. If you are able to wax the hair at this time, do so. (You will find that in most male clients you cannot wax the beard area because the hair follicles are too coarse.) Once you have waxed the area apply a medicated mask designed to absorb oils and encourage healing. After removing the facial mask apply the proper lotion for afterwax care. You may find that you may have to do this procedure with a client who suffers from pseudofolliculitis once a month. Because of all the extra time, special procedures, and products needed to complete this service, you may want to increase your service charge. (3) Ingrown hairs in the leg area as well as the bikini area are common. In the bikini area one or two hairs might become embedded; if this is the case follow step 1 mentioned above. In the case of ingrown hairs on the legs the area is generally larger. When this occurs it is generally due to the top layer of skin growing rapidly over the hair follicle. If you are able to lift the hair prior to waxing, do so. If you find the area too large, explain the situation to the client. Suggest that between waxing the client should use a loofa or a buff puff to slough off dead skin cells. Encourage your client to use the sponges in the opposite direction of hair growth. This procedure should aid in your success in future hair removal procedures. (4) High-frequency current is designed to destroy bacteria. I would suggest using high-frequency current after extraction of a hair follicle from an area that has a red papule, a cyst, or irritation.

Hair Stubble

Occasionally after waxing hair will remain that is too short to grasp the muslin cloth. When this happens, you should send the client home with a clean area. Remember, your goal is to satisfy clients by completing the job they came in for. The following steps will aid you in this situation. This technique should help get your client into a waxing cycle. A first-time client who desires hair removal from the chin and neck may not feel comfortable letting the hair grow for four to six weeks (especially professional, working women). The main objective here is to get the client on a cycle that will enable you to wax the area and remove all the hair within four to six weeks. Follow these steps:

1. First prepare the skin for waxing.

2. Wax the area as usual.

3. Apply wax to three or four hairs only.

4. Take a blunt-edged tweezer, grasp the hair follicle, and pull the hair in the direction of the hair growth. Be sure to keep the tweezer close to the skin. There will be no resistance to the hair being removed from the hair shaft.

5. Continue this procedure until all the hair stubble is removed. The key to the success of this procedure is to apply only a small amount of wax over a few hairs. The warmth of the wax opens up the hair shaft and allows the hair follicle to slide out very easily without breaking the follicle. You will find that the regrowth rate will be the same as the other waxed hair. You may need to inform your client that if she has been shaving, she will find some regrowth of hair. Inform her that any new hair she sees within a few days is the result of shaving and that she should return so you can finish the procedure. This service does require more of your time, and you may want to increase your service charge.

Wax Where You Don't Want It

Quite often in shaping and designing areas to be waxed we place wax where we don't want it. When this happens you should remember that you can only remove hair once the muslin cloth has been placed over the wax. If you find yourself in this situation, the best thing to do is to manipulate the muslin cloth so it does not cover the area where you have mistakenly applied wax. Once you have removed the desired hair you should shape the remaining areas with a tweezer. To remove the undesired wax apply oil to a cloth and wipe the excessive wax off. Wash the area if necessary. The key to remember in avoiding the removal of hair you wish to keep is not to apply muslin cloth over the area!

Hair Growing in Many Different Directions

Hair on underarms, lips, bikini area, and upper thighs in women quite often will grow in different directions. To assure complete hair removal you must treat each hair growth direction separately. An example of this type of procedure is the underarms. The hair could grow in five different directions. If this is the case you should apply wax to each section in the direction of growth and remove the wax in the opposite direction, making sure that you follow the procedure one section at a time. The same will hold true for any face and body waxing. The procedure may seem time consuming; however, when you take the time to do each section correctly from the start you actually save time by avoiding unnecessary corrective steps.

Hair and Wax Left on the Skin

You have applied the wax, covered it with muslin, applied the proper amount of pressure, and snatched the muslin away in the opposite direction, but the hair did not come out, and wax remained on the skin. What went wrong? Ask yourself these questions: (1) Did I pull my muslin cloth in the opposite direction of the hair growth? (2) Is my wax too cold? (Wax was thick, tacky, and did not go on in a thin layer). (3) My choice of muslin is unbleached. When purchasing muslin in bulk be sure the fabric has not been treated with a chemical such as a fabric softener. (4) Is my client's skin damp, cold, or clammy? (If so, be sure to rub a powder over the skin.)

If you do run into a situation where wax remains on the skin you can remove it by reapplying wax over the present wax and applying more pressure on the muslin cloth before removal. This wax application should warm the existing wax, making it softer and easier to remove.

The four waxing situations mentioned above occur with the best of epilators. Knowing how to remedy the situation is very important, especially when a client is present and watching you work. Read over the situations so you can be prepared!

REVIEW QUESTIONS

1. How can you alleviate problems caused by pseudofolliculitis on a male client's face?
2. What steps are used when a client has stubble that needs to be waxed?
3. What measures should the epilator take to ensure that only the desired hairs are removed?
4. If wax remains on the skin after removal of the muslin cloth, what steps could have been missed?

CHAPTER EIGHT

Oops—How
Did I Do That?

CHAPTER OBJECTIVES

1. To inform an epilator of common mistakes that can occur during a waxing procedure

2. To discuss how these incidents occur

3. To discuss solutions to mistakes made during a waxing procedure

I remember a young lady who trained with me for esthetics. We had just had a session on waxing brows and she was waxing a client's brows that afternoon. The salon setup was such that there were eight client positions in one room. The atmosphere was very quiet and peaceful. Four estheticians working on eight clients that afternoon. I will never forget the client scream and demand a mirror! Her shrill voice caused everyone to look up and turn in her direction. The trainee had removed her entire brow! She had placed a used muslin strip back over the client's brow, not knowing that the used area was still strong enough to remove hair. All eventually worked out, but the situation devastated the client as well as the esthetician.

Bruising

Bruising and tenderness are commonly caused errors made by new epilators. Bruising occurs mainly in the bikini and the upper leg area. Most clients will not return to an epilator who caused this discomfort and inconvenience, so it is best to learn how to avoid this painful mistake. Bruising occurs when the epilator does not hold the skin taut. No matter how difficult it may be to reach the area, you must hold the skin in some taut position. You should manipulate your body to achieve the best position to grip the cloth and hold the skin taut to prevent a bruise. You can hold the skin taut in the direction of the hair growth, in the opposite direction, or along the sides of the area to be waxed. You can bruise the skin when you do not pull the muslin cloth close to the skin. If your muslin hand is in the air after pulling the muslin cloth away you can cause a bruise. Look at your hand—is it close to the body being waxed or is it up in the air? Pulling the muslin cloth off too slowly (peeling the cloth off) will also cause bruising and tenderness. You must pull the cloth off quickly while holding the skin taut. I don't know any remedy for bruised skin but time, so the best advice I can give is to hold the skin taut while pulling the muslin cloth quickly!

Burns

Burns are self-explanatory. They are caused when you simply apply wax that is too warm to the client's skin. The client may tell you from the very beginning that she feels discomfort. Remember, every client's tolerance is different. Always pretest your wax. If you are observant, you can tell the difference between skin that is sensitive and skin that has been burned. This is evident from the appearance of the skin. Burned skin will naturally look very red. In some cases it will be obvious that too many layers of skin have been taken away. If you can recognize a burn, it's best to treat it with a burn cream immediately. I would also tell the client that you believe the wax was too warm for the skin and that the client may notice some dark areas in a day or two, or possibly excessive flakiness. Ask the client to inform you of any of these symptoms on the next visit. Admitting that the wax was too warm will demonstrate your creditability and responsibility. On your client's next visit, you should state your intention to adjust the wax to a comfortable temperature. You may even want to offer a complimentary service.

Fine White Pustules

White pustules can occur when you are waxing the face and lip areas. Generally, pustules that appear during waxing are due to overstimulation of the sebaceous glands. Some situations that cause overstimulation of the sebaceous glands are using a muslin strip too large for the area being waxed, failing to use small strips over an area, and not holding the skin taut. Chapter 5 covers individual methods for face and lips, and by following these techniques you can avoid white pustules. If your client complains of fine white bumps, suggest making a compress of baking soda and water (1 tablespoon of baking soda to a pint of water) and applying it to the area. The disincrustation solution should emulsify the oils and dry them more quickly. When waxing the face or the lip area in some clients it is better to use small strips and do small sections. You will find this to be true with sensitive clients and those with active sebaceous glands.

Removed Too Much Hair?

When waxing brows be sure you examine the shape of the brows thoroughly to make sure this is the shape you desire before applying the muslin cloth. If you still remove too much hair ask yourself a few questions: (1) Did you apply too much wax, so that when you applied pressure to adhere the cloth to the wax, it spread to an undesired area? (2) Did you use a used muslin strip? When waxing the brow or the lip use the muslin strip only once. When you have used a strip once, throw it away! To avoid unnecessary mistakes, remember, when it comes to face, lip, and brows, use the muslin strip once and throw it away! (3) Is your wax area free from wax that may have dropped from towels, sheets, head wraps etc.? (4) Are your hands and fingers free from wax? (5) Did you measure the brow shape correctly? (6) Is your wax stick dripping wax?

This example involves eyebrows, but the same questions can be asked about any area you are attempting to wax.

We have covered common first-time mistakes. By being aware of these errors you may be able to avoid them. If you do find yourself in one of these situations, remember, you will only make the mistake once.

REVIEW QUESTIONS

1. What is the major cause of bruising, and how can it be avoided?

2. If fine white pustules appear after waxing an area, what treatment can be applied?

3. How do you prevent burns on a client's skin?

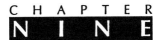

CHAPTER
NINE

Buzzwords

CHAPTER OBJECTIVES

1. To discuss alternative waxing techniques available

2. To introduce the epilator to various advanced products on the market

3. To discuss the difference between speedwaxing and the standard procedure

The saying that the world keeps getting smaller is so true. What seems new to us may have existed for a long time. This is true in waxing. Banding, European, and speedwaxing are waxing methods that have now become the esthetic industry buzzwords. Specialized training is required for each of these services. You can learn each technique by attending conferences that offer small, individualized classes. I would also recommend that you gain command of the standard methods of waxing first because they pose their own problems that need to be mastered. But as a novice you should expand your mind and learn all that you can. Let's review these different techniques, and maybe you will find one that appeals to you.

Banding

Banding is a method of hair removal that comes from the Middle East as well as the ancient Orient. The technique uses only a string! You can wax legs, arms, brows, etc. with just a string. A piece of string is held in the mouth, and a loop is made at the bottom of the string, tying the ends together. The ends are twisted so that movement is allowed. The string is then placed on the area to be waxed and the string is twisted to grasp the hair, pulling the hair out of the root. The epilator who masters these techniques can remove hair as quickly as with standard waxing procedure. Banding is now being promoted by the esthetic industry because of new skin technologies. Retin A, gycolic acids, and cosmetic surgery make the skin sensitive to depilatory waxing. An epilator who can diversify and switch to banding to service a client is one who will have a great deal of credibility.

Speedwaxing

Speedwaxing is a method of waxing that speeds the waxing procedure. I only recommend practicing this method after you have mastered the standard methods. When applying wax in speedwaxing the epilator divides the leg into two sections, top and bottom. Cover the entire lower half of the leg with wax before removing with a muslin strip. You then apply a muslin strip to the wax (strips are standard size for leg waxing) smooth, and pull in the opposite direction quickly. In the same stroke reapply the cloth over the next section of wax, smooth, and pull back in the opposite direction. Continue in that manner until the entire lower leg is waxed. Follow the same procedure with the upper portion of the leg. Turn the client over and follow the same procedure on the back of the legs. The difference in this technique is that you move so quickly that you apply the wax all at once before reaching for the muslin strip. You do not apply one strip of wax and then remove that one strip. You do not stop to reapply wax, you do not change strips, and do not tap the skin until all one section is waxed. How is this type of method better than the standard? Clients feel that the quicker the hair is removed the better. The usual time needed to wax legs with the standard method is approximately forty minutes; speedwaxing takes fifteen to twenty minutes. The entire bikini area, upper leg, and lower leg can be accomplished in thirty-five minutes!

Again, the key to speedwaxing is to cover the entire divided section with wax, then remove the hair with one muslin strip. The trained epilator can determine when to discard the strip by the weight and the sound of the pull. I would advise those who desire to learn speedwaxing to attend a class or get an experienced epilator to teach you how to accomplish this technique.

European Waxing

European waxing involves waxing without using a muslin strip. This wax method is sometimes called the cold wax procedure or the green wax method. The wax used is a different formula than that of a honey wax, and the wax can be applied by hand or with a spatula. You should test the wax to be sure of the proper temperature. After applying the wax you should check for the proper cooling. The wax should be pliable when touched, and when the wax has cooled slightly you grasp the edge of the wax and quickly pull it in the opposite direction of hair growth. The wax can be reused—heated, filtered, and then reused. You can reuse the wax repeatedly before replacing it with fresh wax. With the importance of sanitation today, however, many epilators prefer to discard the wax. The cold wax method has the advantage that buying muslin is not necessary. It is also said to be quicker than the standard method. The main difference between the cold wax method and the European method is that cold wax can cool to the point of turning hard. In the European method or green wax method the wax stays pliable and can be reapplied to the next area before returning it to be reheated. This method really increases your speed. After seeing a demonstration of the European green wax method many epilators are willing to give it a try.

The best way to appreciate these methods is to watch them in action. I watch for listings of classes or demonstrations in any literature that announces classes in advance.

REVIEW QUESTIONS

1. When can the technique of banding be used?
2. What feature is unique about green wax?
3. Explain the difference between speedwaxing and the standard procedure.
4. The beginning epilator should master what technique first? Why?

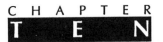

C H A P T E R
T E N

Marketing Depilatory Waxing

CHAPTER OBJECTIVES

1. To show how and why waxing is a profitable service for an esthetician's salon

2. To discuss ways to advertise and increase business

Waxing can be one of the most profitable of all esthetic services. This statement is based on the amount of materials needed to wax an area and the length of time it takes to accomplish the job. A good example of this is waxing the brow. It takes approximately twenty minutes to wax brows. The cost of materials is estimated to be twenty cents! The charge for the service ten to fifteen dollars. If you wax three brows in an hour you would make thirty dollars for one hour, with a cost of materials of sixty cents. That's a great profit!

I often hear estheticians say that the summer months are slow months. But I know estheticians who have higher paychecks because of increased business due to waxing. Once you have mastered your waxing skills and start to receive compliments, you should start advertising your service. A great way to advertise is to give services away. If your client is in your salon to receive another service, give her a waxing service at no charge. Once she tries your service, she will have to return to receive it again. If your skills are good she will refer others to you. Have a keen eye. Recommend your services as you see clients who need them.

While you are waxing one area, ask if your client has tried waxing in other areas. Take the time to explain the benefits of the service. Most clients are not aware of all the areas that can be waxed and their benefits.

Advertising in the Salon

Your salon is the best place to advertise. You can hang a poster that displays a particular summer waxing item, for instance lower legs or bikini area.

If you have a boutique in your area that sells swimwear ask if you can leave some flyers. A better marketing technique would be to offer a complimentary service of bathing suit hair removal with a purchase.

Two for one is an excellent way to introduce another service. With this marketing technique, the client pays for one service and receives another free.

Programs are often a great way to get your client to commit to waxing services, and they provide cash flow. A waxing program usually gives the client six waxing services for the price of five. Another option is to give the client a price discount with the purchase of six services. To enhance the package, include a free service like a facial or a haircut. This way you can introduce a new service the salon is offering.

List the special of the month on a poster. Place it where clients have to wait before services. Make sure your services and specials are listed in the windows and easily seen by those passing by.

Marketing Outside the Salon

Marketing outside the salon area can bring new business to you and for your salon. Take literature to modeling agencies, photographers, doctors, and health spas. If you have the opportunity to speak at community centers, groups, or organizations, demonstrate waxing the brows. The effect of working on one of the group members and improving her appearance by reshaping her brows to a more youthful appearance will create excitement and ensure future business.

Marketing is one of the most beneficial steps you can take to increase your business and to promote your services. Word-of-mouth is the best form of advertisement. If you remember to give, give, give away you will find that the investment of your time will bring you a healthy return. A free service is really never free if you have a good eye.

One quick hand, another one taut, and good word-of-mouth advertising will bring you a very successful career . . . . Hairs to you!

CHAPTER QUESTIONS

1. Why is waxing so profitable for an esthetician?
2. What is one of the best ways to advertise?
3. What are other ways to market your business?

Answers to Review Questions

Chapter 1

1. Why is depilatory waxing so popular?

It is a quick, simple, convenient, and affordable procedure. It is ideal for any size area that needs to be waxed. It can be used on sensitive and delicate areas. All the hair can be removed in one visit. Waxing also removes the right amount of dead skin. And, finally, it takes up to four to six weeks for the hair to grow back before the procedure needs to be repeated.

2. In addition to depilatory waxing, what are some other methods of hair removal?

There are many different hair removal methods, including shaving, tweezing, chemical depilatories, and electrolysis.

3. Describe the structure of the hair.

The hair develops within the follicle. At the bottom of the follicle is the papilla, which supplies blood to the cells. The follicle is surrounded by involuntary muscles, which, when contracted, press on the sebaceous glands, which in turn release sebum to lubricate the skin.

4. What are some factors a client must consider before choosing electrolysis?

The person administering electrolysis must be certified and highly trained. The procedure is also very uncomfortable, and it can take one to three years to destroy hair from large areas. In addition, this procedure is very expensive.

Chapter 2

1. What is the purpose of prewax products?

Prewax products help remove dampness or oils on the area that is to be waxed.

2. What is the difference between soft wax and cold wax?

Soft wax requires using a muslin strip; cold wax does not.

3. What is the suggested size for brow, chin, and leg strips?

Brow strips should be 1 $^1/_2$ by 4 inches; chin strips should be 2 by 4 inches; and leg strips should be 4 by 9 inches.

4. Why should disposable products be considered?

Disposable products will ensure good sanitation practices and can easily be thrown away.

5. What product is considered the most practical spatula?

The tongue suppressor is considered the most practical spatula because it can be cut to fit the needs of the epilator and in addition, is disposable.

Chapter 3

1. What source should the epilator turn to for sterilization and sanitation requirements?

    The epilator should consult the state's board, which governs the cosmetology and esthetics profession.

2. Why should the epilator wear gloves?

    Although it is a personal choice, the epilator should wear gloves to avoid infection, especially if there is an open cut or wound present.

3. What is the best way to sterilize waxing implements?

    To sterilize waxing implements, wash them with a bacterial soap, immerse them in a disinfectant solution for twenty minutes, and store them in a cabinet containing Formalin.

4. What should the epilator's attitude be about maintaining the facility?

    Epilators should ask if they would be willing to lie on the bed, place their heads on the pillow, and have the implements used on their faces. If the answer is no, then the epilator should do what is necessary to improve the sanitation and sterilization of the facility so that the epilator, as well as the client, would feel comfortable and safe having a waxing service.

Chapter 4

1. What are the five basic waxing steps?

    The five basic waxing steps are (1) the application of the wax, (2) holding the skin taut, (3) removal of the wax, (4) position of the cloth when pulled, and (5) tapping and slapping after the cloth is pulled.

2. How should the temperature of the wax be tested?

   The temperature of the wax is tested by monitoring the heater gauge, by observing the flow of wax, and by feeling the consistency of the wax.

3. What step should be done before the waxing begins?

   The client's hair should be trimmed before the waxing begins.

4. What five points should be considered when starting the waxing procedure?

   Five points should be considered when starting the waxing procedure, including what the client desires to be done, the objective of the procedure, the area to be waxed, whether the area was properly prepared, and whether the strip is the correct size.

5. Why is it important to control the wax?

   The wax must be controlled to prevent the procedure from becoming messy and creating unnecessary problems.

Chapter 5

1. Name three important factors to keep in mind when waxing the brows, lips, bikini area, and facial hair.

   Keep in mind that only a small amount of wax should be used, the hair should be trimmed, and the skin should be kept taut while waxing.

2. What is the goal of the waxing procedure?

The goal of waxing is to remove all of the hair without needing to tweeze more than five hairs.

3. After waxing a client's back, what steps are taken to ease discomfort?

After waxing a client's back, apply a towel compress that has been soaked in a solution of baking soda and water.

Chapter 6

1. How does a solution of baking soda and water help if there is discomfort after waxing?

Baking soda and water help emulsify oils, remove the redness, and calm skin irritation.

2. What equipment is used after waxing facial hairs?

High-frequency equipment is very effective for destroying bacteria and preventing the possibility of cysts.

3. What should be done after finishing a waxing procedure?

After a waxing procedure, remove any wax residue, apply aftercare astringent, and finally apply a calming protection lotion.

4. What product is used to reduce irritation caused by friction after waxing?

Use powder after the protection lotion to reduce friction after waxing.

Chapter 7

1. How can you alleviate problems caused by pseudo-folliculitis on a male client's face?

   Before waxing a male client's face that has pseudo-folliculitis, tweeze the ingrown hair out first, do a facial to prepare the skin for epilation, and then proceed with the waxing procedure.

2. What steps are used when a client has stubble that needs to be waxed?

   When there is stubble that needs to be removed, apply a small amount of wax to a few hairs of the stubble and remove the hair with tweezers.

3. What measures should the epilator take to ensure that only the desired hairs are removed?

   The epilator can ensure that only the desired hairs will be waxed by not putting wax where it shouldn't be.

4. If wax remains on the skin after removal of the muslin cloth, what steps could have been missed?

   If wax remains on the skin after the muslin is pulled, it is possible that the wax was too cold, the cloth was not pulled in the opposite direction of hair growth, the client's skin was cold or clammy, or the muslin used had been treated with chemicals like fabric softeners.

Chapter 8

1. What is the major cause of bruising, and how can it be avoided?

   Bruising is caused when the skin is not held taut. Always hold the skin taut when waxing.

2. If fine white pustules appear after waxing an area, what treatment can be applied?

A solution of baking soda and water can be applied to an area that develops white pustules. This solution will emulsify the oils due to overstimulation of the sebaceous glands.

3. How do you prevent burns on a client's skin?

Burns can be prevented by testing the wax and making sure the wax is not too hot before it is applied to the client's skin.

Chapter 9

1. When can the technique of banding be used?

Banding is used for clients who have sensitive skin due to Retin A, gycolic acids, cosmetic surgery, or other conditions.

2. What feature is unique about green wax?

Green wax is unique in that it can be reheated and reused.

3. Explain the difference between speedwaxing and the standard procedure.

In the speedwaxing procedure, wax is applied all at the same time before the muslin is used and is completed in about half the time of the standard procedure.

4. The beginning epilator should master what technique first? Why?

The beginning epilator should master the standard procedure to gain speed and expertise. Speed waxing requires a secure and steady hand.

Chapter 10

1. Why is waxing so profitable for an esthetician?

   Waxing is profitable because it requires a minimal amount of supplies and very little time.

2. What is one of the best ways to advertise?

   Giving a free or complimentary service to a client who is in for a different service is one of the best forms of advertising. If the client likes the free service, she'll come back for more, and will probably tell her friends!

3. What are other ways to market your business?

   Other ways to market your business include displaying posters that promote your services or specials that are running, leaving flyers with various vendors in the neighborhood, offering two-for-one services, or offering a discount for buying a certain number of services.